HOSPITAL FINANCE

A Comprehensive Case Approach

Jerry L. Bolandis

St. Elizabeth Medical Center
Granite City, Illinois

St. Louis University
St. Louis, Missouri

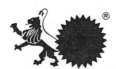

AN ASPEN PUBLICATION®
Aspen Systems Corporation
Rockville, Maryland
London
1982

Library of Congress Cataloging in Publication Data

Bolandis, Jerry L.
Hospital finance.

Includes bibliographies and index.
1. Hospitals—Finance. 2. Hospitals—
Finance—Case studies. I. Title.
RA971.3.B64   362.1'1'0681   81-20506
ISBN: 0-89443-377-6   AACR2

Library of Congress Catalog Card Number: 81-20506
ISBN: 0-89443-377-6

Printed in the United States of America

1   2   3   4   5

To my Mom,
the memory of my Dad,
my wife, Janet,
and my children, Beth, Matt, and Brooke

Table of Contents

Preface

The purpose of this book is to present not only the theoretical aspects of health care finance but also the practical application of these theories to managerial decision making in the health care institution. It is essential that the student of health care finance understand the application of basic principles to a real-life setting and interrelate effectively with the environment in which the manager operates both internally and externally with the institution. Thus, the text explores basic finance concepts with direct application to a real world case that extends throughout the book. In many instances, of course, in making managerial decisions there may be no real answers. Accordingly, the work is based on the premise that decisions are made within an organized framework and based on the most current information available.

The book's organization follows the components of the financial cycle: (1) reporting, (2) action, (3) planning, and (4) control. However, these segments cannot be divorced from each other; they are completely integrated, with many of them occurring concurrently. It must also be emphasized that the health care institution operates within a very complex and dynamic environment that includes governmental regulation, patient relations, and physician interactions. In this context, in the institution's daily operations, the most important aspects of the health care environment, the patient and the quality of the care provided are sometimes overlooked.

The author hopes to provide insights into the operations of health care facilities from a finance viewpoint and to provide theoretical tools that financial managers and administrators can use and adapt to their particular circumstances. However, it should be stressed that the case study presented here provides only one example of such an operation; it is not intended to be taken as the perfect model. There is always room for learning and improvements.

The material presented in this text is illustrative of current topics of interest. Because of the dynamic nature of the field, readers should research individual projects before taking specific action.

J.L.B.

Acknowledgments

Numerous persons have had a part in the development of this book. I would particularly like to acknowledge the contributions of those persons who have influenced greatly my work in the health care field. First, I would like to thank the staff and board members of St. Elizabeth Medical Center, Granite City, Illinois, for providing me with the opportunity to be a part of such an organization. I would like to acknowledge those persons at Arthur Andersen with whom I have associated in their audit capacity at St. Elizabeth Medical Center. I would also like to thank the faculty of St. Louis University, particularly Dr. Richard Fox and Dr. Thomas Dolan, for giving me the opportunity to participate in the instruction of M.H.A. students. I also extend my thanks to the students of the M.H.A. program at St. Louis University for their interest in the field of health care administration and finance.

I extend my deepest thanks to my family for their patience and understanding. I cannot adequately repay the dedication of my Mom and Dad, Gerda and Albert Bolandis, who taught me the value of education and the fundamental principles of work that have inspired the respect and basic ideals on which my work and life are based. I hope that I have at least a portion of their dedication.

Finally, but not least important, is the strength provided me by my wife, Janet L. (Yeager) Bolandis, and my three children, Beth Ann, Matthew James, and Brooke Alison. Without their support and understanding, this book would have been impossible.

References to any real persons or institutions are purely coincidental. The material presented in the case study is fictional. I take full responsibility for the content of this text; those mentioned here have no share in this responsibility.

Part I

Introduction

The purpose of this section is to introduce the reader to the hospital finance environment. One cannot be limited to strict accounting theories as applied to the hospital industry and hope to achieve effectiveness in dealing with a unique and pressure-filled environment. Thus, this first part will deal with the hospital environment in general and then move on to the specific case. A frame of reference in finance will be established to initiate the reader's involvement in the case study, which will illustrate the theories discussed throughout the text.

Chapter 1 deals with the basic organization of the hospital and the environment in which it operates. Specific reference is made to the increasing need for sound financial management and for specific definitions of the financial duties and responsibilities in the financial cycle. Key financial pressures in today's environment are the result of the balancing of increased technology and demands for "better" patient care with reductions or containments in cost. Basic philosophies related to universally sound fiscal management—return on investment, financial planning, and cost effectiveness—are somewhat new to an industry based on providing the best possible care to those in need regardless of the cost or the ability of the individual to finance the services received.

Chapter 2 introduces the reader to the case-study hospital, which will provide the frame of reference for applying the various theories. The hospital, Community Medical Center, is a 350-bed, acute care facility located in a midwestern, urban environment. It is the sole provider in a primary service area of about 100,000 people. The percentages of Medicare and Medicaid utilization have increased steadily in the past several years, and alternative sources of revenue are the primary focus of the hospital's administration.

Beyond the basic outline of the case hospital, a secondary aspect focuses on the basic organizational philosophies and practices related to the finance function. In the context of the theories presented, readers will be asked to compare their views and philosophies of management with those illustrated in the case study. In this way, direct reader involvement will be facilitated.

It is important to note that hospital costs are really charges to Medicare and many Medicaid and Blue Cross programs. Thus, the terms *costs* and *charges* are often used interchangeably in the examination of the inflationary costs of health care. Finally, while the theories of health-care inflation presented in this section are based on economic theory, the detailed analysis is the author's. It is hoped that readers will find the presentation thought-provoking in formulating their own opinions on the economics of present health-care delivery systems.

Chapter 1

The Role and Environment of Current Hospital Finance

INTRODUCTION

The purpose of this chapter is to provide readers with an environmental frame of reference for examining present health care systems, particularly hospital delivery systems. To achieve this, it is necessary to present and comment on some suggested causes of inflation in health care systems. In considering these causes, readers are left to develop their own frames of economic reference; detailed economic analysis of these aspects lies outside the scope of the present work.

Throughout this discussion, as noted earlier, reference is made to cost inflation as synonymous with inflation of charges in a cost reimbursement system such as Medicare. While this may be somewhat confusing in analyzing an inflation that is usually identified with charges in hospitals, the distinction between costs and charges has in practice become blurred, given present cost reimbursement practices.

HISTORICAL DEVELOPMENTS

As we enter the 1980s, the health care delivery system in the United States must be regarded with awe as one of the most technologically advanced systems in the world. Historically, the general populace has required and demanded the most sophisticated treatments and research for known ailments. Hospitals in particular were at the forefront in the development and acquisition of the facilities and equipment that were believed to be the most effective in treating disease and trauma. This leadership role was founded on the basic philosophy of better patient care and the attraction and retention of the most qualified physicians available. Very little thought was given to the cost effectiveness of such acquisitions or to the availability of alternative sources in the immediate area. Competition therefore focused on quality rather than cost. This attitude was fueled by the growth of third party payers as insurance became available to the general population.

As facilities grew and became more complex, cost increases compounded at a dramatic rate. The inception of Medicare and Medicaid in the mid-1960s as historic cost reimbursement programs did little to curtail the spiral of inflation in the health care sector. The benefits of insurance coverage via these programs to the aged, disabled, and poor increased utilization of health care facilities to such an extent that federal funds were made available through the Hill-Burton Program to finance the construction of new and expanded facilities for the delivery of care. As the costs increased to the government through Medicare and Medicaid, various theories were advanced to explain the reasons behind the dramatic increases in hospital costs and charges.

Today, health care delivery in the United States accounts for over $90 billion in expenditures each year with an annual growth rate of 10 to 14 percent. There are over 7,100 hospitals with about 1.6 million beds and over $40 billion in assets. The number of hospital employees has increased from about 800 thousand in 1946 to over 3 million at the present time. Given these statistics, it is little wonder that health care delivery has become the focus of attention.

CAUSES OF HEALTH CARE INFLATION

There are at least ten theories that have been advanced to explain the causes of health care inflation:

1. Demand-pull
2. Cost-push
3. Overinvestment
4. Technological imperative
5. Overconsumption
6. Supply creates demand (Say's law)
7. Monopoly
8. Physician as consumer
9. Demographic
10. System-induced

Demand-Pull

The demand-pull explanation has its theoretical base in the effects of increased demand with a smaller shift in supply. Many have argued that the implementation of Medicare and Medicaid have resulted in upward thrusts of demand that have yet to be met by supply. On a macro scale, increased demand resulted from these programs as health services (particularly hospitalization and physician services) became available to the poor and aged segments of the general public. In certain areas—particularly in communities serviced by a single provider and a limited number of physicians—increased demand has undoubtedly resulted in the need for expansion of both capital and labor. However, one cannot place the entire burden on increased demand. Current statistics indicate that on any given day, 15 to 20 percent of hospital beds are empty, with few hospitals experiencing an average of 90 percent occupancy or higher. Physicians also have increased in relative numbers, but this is only a manifestation of Say's law that stipulates that supply generates demand. Based on these facts, demand-pull does not appear to be at the root of the inflation in health care.

Cost-Push

A somewhat more realistic description of medical care inflation is cost-push. In this theory, suppliers increase costs, which are passed through to the consumer (patient). With resources expanded to cover cost increases to an everincreasing extent, this theory appears to embrace all the proposed explanations of rising health care costs. Physicians and hospitals have an almost unlimited resource base for accumulating the reserves required to cover costs. This is possible because of the "zero price" created by third party payers, whether private or governmental. The illusion of an unlimited resource base has been capitalized on by hospitals in setting rates higher in heavily used third party areas, for example, in room rates, laboratory, and radiology, which are heavily covered by third party payments, while keeping charges lower and costs down in the emergency room and outpatient areas that are covered by little third party participation. Cost reimbursement has done little to curtail costs, but it has given providers an incentive to adjust rates and purchases to maximize this reimbursement. Indeed, in recent bond issues there is usually a covenant in the indenture that replacements or capital acquisitions be at a high enough level that depreciation reimbursement will not deteriorate over say the 20- to 30-year life of the bonds. Unless a total change in reimbursement and modes of delivering health care services is forthcoming, it would appear that inflation in the health care sector will continue at the same pace or even at a more rapid rate in the future.

Overinvestment

The overinvestment theory postulates that the medical sector has invested in capital resources to an extent beyond what can be utilized on an efficient basis. The costs of underutilized services are passed on via higher costs for those utilized services. This is a valid factor, but it can be encompassed by cost-push theory. Providers are continuously "enhancing" services that often "cannibalize" existing procedures. In general, discontinuing or sharing underutilized services is rare among providers. The recent emphasis on outpatient care has resulted only in adding outpatient facilities and service areas in conjunction with inpatient services and facilities, leading to higher overall charges and cost reimbursement claims.

Technological Imperative

Tied in with the above explanation is the theory that physicians are taken up with technology and technological improvements regardless of the costs or benefits. Continually enhancing services and technology serves merely to reduce utilization in existing methodologies of treatment and diagnosis. This is in line with both the overinvestment and the cost-push theories.

Overconsumption and Say's Law

Overconsumption and the fact that supply creates demand appear to be closely related as a root cause of the failure to establish a mechanism to moderate health care expenditures. Prices that generally control access to goods and services are not apparent to consumers of medical services; therefore, everyone seeks the most (quantity) available (supply). This operates to allow physicians and hospitals to increase costs and charges without affecting demand and to increase the variety of treatment methodologies, which almost always have users.

Monopoly and Physicians as Consumers

The proposition that providers act as a national monopoly and that physicians are consumers fits into this picture. Consumers rarely compare prices for medical care; rather they rely heavily on their physicians to order appropriate tests and treatments, often, the more technical, the better. Physicians demand increased technology and services that the hospitals are willing, indeed, almost forced, to provide, given the medical market's reliance on physician demand and the few incentives to cut costs or charges. Again, the theoretical base for this is in cost-push, where providers naturally upgrade services and technology at increased costs, which apparently keeps everyone happy in the maze of relations between patient, physician, hospital, third party payer, and employer.

Demographic

There is some merit in the theory that, because we have made services available to the poor and aged and because the population is increasing in age and in the complexity of disease patterns, health care is shifting to the longer and more chronic forms of illness that require custodial care and lengthy interaction with health care providers. This may explain some of the increases, yet providers have generally met the needs of these groups within existing service provisions and capabilities. If anything, providers have sought increased revenue by providing "specialized" services to these groups. This has resulted in further duplication and underutilization of existing service facilities.

System-Induced

In fact, the system is the real culprit in health care inflation. The picture painted above points to an inefficient, cost-ineffective mode of delivering health care to the public. As long as we have cost reimbursement, makeshift planning efforts and provide few incentives to curtail costs, health care inflation will continue in the guise of enhanced patient care.

REDUCING HEALTH CARE COSTS

There are several factors to be considered in any proposal to alleviate the strain of the existing delivery system's cost increases. First, arbitrary caps are not the means to solve the problem. With this method, too many necessary services in efficiently operated facilities may suffer. However, area limits on the total available to charge per capita should be implemented with local agencies who are charged with the allocation process on a prospective, area-wide basis. Second, allowing providers to keep excess reimbursement will provide incentives to control physicians and to establish a health maintenance organization (HMO) philosophy in delivering health care services. Third, all categories of providers must be included. It does no good to include hospitals and physicians and exclude nursing homes. Finally, steps should be taken to document cost-benefit analyses of services based on a sociological perspective. Funds will continue to be allocated subjectively and services will increasingly be provided at random unless some effort is made to determine the benefits and costs to the public within particular areas.

In summary, the examination of the various descriptive theories of inflation in the health care sector leads to the conclusion that the system is at the root of the problem. Within the system, the most significant individual cause of inflation in the health care sector appears to be that postulated by the cost-push theory. Providers have few incentives to contain cost, but they have many incentives to move up the average cost curve and to realize higher revenues without any viable cost containment measures. The only solutions appear to be a revamping of the modes of delivery and a refinement of the reimbursement system to encourage, perhaps even force, cost-effective and efficient behavior.

These solutions are not easily implemented. Many proposals have been introduced to attack particular aspects of the inflation problem: mandatory cost and charge limits, prospective rate reviews, limits on capital spending, area planning via Health Systems Agencies (HSAs), routine cost limits on Medicare reimbursement, and numerous containment programs attached to national health insurance proposals. Hospitals have responded to these containment pressures via the existing Voluntary Effort Program. Inflation under this program has been reduced to a manageable level. The conclusion must be that, given the motivation to do so, the hospital industry is capable of controlling itself. As a single industry in an inflationary environment, however, it cannot hope to reduce its inflation below the levels of the environment in which it operates. Placing cost caps on one segment of the economy can only lead to reduced levels of services as the normal costs of daily operations rise.

While cost containment is a primary concern in today's environment, there are other environmental factors that affect hospital costs. Hospitals in general have historically been concerned primarily with direct matching revenue and expense on a historical cost basis. Medicare, Blue Cross, and, in most cases, Medicaid reimburse hospitals for historical costs only, not allowing for any profit to 501(c)(3) (not-for-profit) hospitals and allowing a minimal return to for-profit institutions. Historically, and far too frequently now, hospitals have planned for current operating expenses and matched these expenses with rates and contributions to cover only these short-term projections. Charges have been paid almost without question by insurance companies, leading the insured patient to believe that hospital costs were minimal at best. The current emphasis on cost reductions and reductions in the level of philanthropy has limited the revenue-generating capacity of hospitals. As historical cost reimbursement grows and inflation continues, the average hospital is faced with a lack of funds suitable for asset replacement and with fewer funds available for technological enhancements. Consequently, hospitals are faced with substantial amounts of debt, the servicing of which places additional inflationary pressures on the provision of hospital services.

In addition to being adversely affected by planning deficiencies, the health care field is becoming increasingly specialized in personnel and must meet regulatory agency standards, such as those of the Joint Commission on Hospital Accreditation (JCHA), in adding these personnel to their staffs. As a general rule, the increase in professionalism and specialization results in higher wage scales and a reduction in productivity, which drive up costs of providing services.

One cannot argue against increased patient care quality, but goals must be set and a medium achieved to maintain quality without allowing productivity to suffer. Staffing patterns must be justified in the light of productivity standards, which are just beginning to be developed in the hospital industry. Increasing emphasis is being placed on tying utilization statistics to financial data on a national scale in order to measure the efficiency of individual hospitals. This emphasis has manifested itself in the proposed Annual Hospital Report (AHR), which has as its basis the movement from the traditional responsibility of accumulation of revenues and expenses to a functional accumulation of costs by service.

A significant environmental factor affecting hospital operations relates to the planning requirements dictated by Public Law 93–641, which established HSAs and certificates of need at the state level. These agencies and planning boards require hospitals to begin the development of long-range service and financial plans that are essential to the area and hospital planning activities. The required planning process must demonstrate service needs as well as economic justifications of cost effectiveness. Shared service alternatives are generally required. These require individual hospitals to develop a cooperative stance in the provision of health care services to their service areas.

Finally, daily operations must be maintained at a level consistent with the overall philosophies of the hospital in the provision of care to those in need. The daily operations must be handled in the most cost-effective manner possible while maintaining the integrity of the services provided. All of the above pressures come to bear on the hospital executives who must deal with the issues and maintain an advantage to maximize their hospitals' positions in the delivery of quality care to those served. The next step is to develop the fiscal philosophies that will guide the hospital into the future.

FISCAL PHILOSOPHIES

As can be seen in the above discussion, the hospital administrator and fiscal officer must consider seriously the financial implications of almost all decisions and actions. The daily operations of the facility must be well-planned and developed to maintain fiscal viability in the dynamic environment in which the facility operates. It is absolutely essential that the chief financial officer maintain financial operations in the organization at a level of priority in keeping with the importance of finance in the hospital industry.

Expanding upon this point, organizational charts of two hospitals are presented in Figure 1–1 for comparative analysis. For present purposes, the graphic representations presented for the two hospitals, Community 1 and Community 2, ignore possible personnel circumstances related to informal organizational operations. With respect to the organizational positioning of fiscal services, a visual comparison of the two charts indicates a functional assignment of duties in line with traditional functional expertise at the administrative level for Community 2. In Community 1, the span of control may be an issue since the executive vice-president is directly responsible for both the nursing and financial functions. Depending on the particular circumstances involved, the structure exhibited by Community 1 does not appear conducive to top-level input into the decision-making process. The structure of Community 2 provides a functional division of duties and span of responsibility that may lead to effective and efficient interaction at the administrative level.[1]

Administrative decisions should lead to those actions that can deal most effectively with the hospital's environmental pressures. To achieve cost efficiencies in daily operations, the hospital administration must develop an action-oriented financial plan that deals not only with short-range objectives, but which also sets the long-range goals that guide the organization through a seven- to ten-year planning period.

While the basic philosophy of setting objectives and planning for the future sounds simplistic, its importance is underscored by the fact of capital erosion, resulting in an increased need for borrowing. No longer can the hospital be complacent about its approach to capital accumulation and to the establishment and achievement of rates of return. Fiscal viability and institutional survival mandate capital accumulation at a rate at least equal to the current inflation rate.

An adequate return can be achieved in any of several ways. However, each method must be directed by top management and be set in the basic philosophies of the organization. Simply raising rates or a complacent reliance on contributions to achieve this objective will be inappropriate at best. A matching of revenues and expenses that focuses on cost effectiveness is the soundest policy a hospital can adopt. To maintain control of financial operations, the hospital administration should adopt a comprehensive framework that will guide the financial operations of the hospital through the financial cycle.

THE FINANCIAL CYCLE

The financial cycle is a continuous process of planning, reporting, action, and control, as illustrated in Figure 1–2. Continuous evaluation and interaction between the phases of the cycle are essential in the dynamics of the

Figure 1-1 Comparative Organizational Charts of Two Hospitals

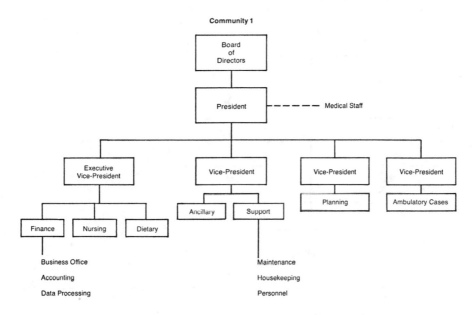

Community 1

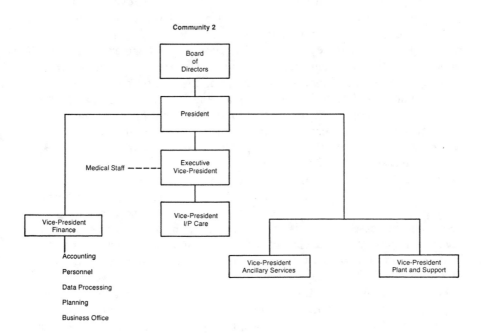

Community 2

Figure 1-2 The Financial Cycle

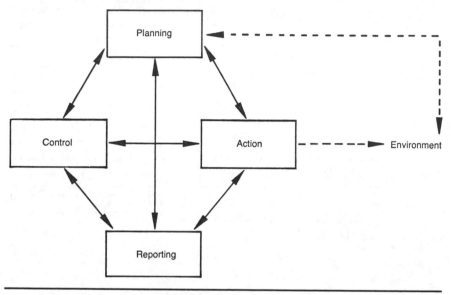

hospital's interaction with its environment. Contingency planning and alternative methods of adaptive action must be a part of the cycle.

The development of the components in each phase of the cycle will be examined in detail in the remaining sections of this book. Part II covers the reporting section of the cycle. Basically, reporting is handled via the traditional accounting functions that relate to the accurate, timely summarization and reporting of the financial operations of the institution. While a basic level of understanding of accounting is assumed in the present work, there are significant alterations in basic industrial accounting as applied to the hospital accounting system. The reporting functions of an institution must be concerned not only with the accurate preparation of accounting data but also with the incorporation of activity data that are essential for effective management of the institution. In the development of hospital accounting in Part II, each classification of accounts is analyzed for its implications in hospital accounting. Contractual allowances, increased use of fund accounting concepts, and increased emphasis on receivables management are some of the areas of utmost importance in the hospital accounting and reporting system. The issues and theories in the reporting section are illustrated in the Community Medical Center case study.

Part III discusses the application of financial and managerial decision making in interaction with key elements of the hospital's financial environment. Selected key elements in the hospital environment must be understood in basic terms so that these elements, which are pervasive in a hospital's effectiveness, can be dealt with as efficiently as possible. Topics of discussion relate to both the internal and external pressures that must be brought under the hospital's control if fiscal viability is to be maintained. These topics are concerned with the action phase of the financial cycle. The word "action" is in fact descriptive of a hospital's way of dealing with its particular environment and internal circumstances. The hospital executive can no longer be complacent in dealing with the hospital's environment. The executive must maintain a posture of action planning to maximize the hospital's position in its particular circumstances. Only with a complete understanding of the key elements that constrain the hospital's actions can the executive develop strategies that will allow the hospital to determine its own destiny.

The third component of the financial cycle is planning. This is the topic of Part IV. The development of both long-range and short-term projections rests on a foundation established by the decisions of top management. Financial inputs into these decisions are discussed in the chapters on forecasting statistics, cost analysis, rate of return, rate setting, and summarization/modeling. Here, a distinction must be drawn between fixed and flexible budgeting. Emphasis is placed on the development of a flexible budget as the most effective model in dealing with the contingencies inherent in the hospital environment. The hospital case study is used to illustrate key issues critical to the planning process. Planning must be viewed as one of the most crucial aspects of financial management. The entire institution is involved in the provision of patient care and in the achievement of hospital objectives. Consequently, it is logical to provide for institution-wide involvement in the planning process. Departmental managers as well as physicians and board members must be included in the process to project reasonable and effective goal levels for the future operations of the entire institution. A secondary benefit of total hospital involvement accrues from the accountability and increased assumption of responsibility by those persons who have direct input into the decision making process.

The final aspect of the financial cycle, that of control, is discussed in Part V. The control phase is necessary to provide feedback to the decision makers in order that corrective or adaptive actions can be taken. The basis of financial control is in the comparative analyses that utilize actual data versus planned performance or trend data over time. Comparative analysis of detailed relationships is essential to the evaluation process. Inherent in control is the adequate reporting of essential information. The data available in a hospital usually overwhelm decision makers in terms of volume, duplication, and conflicting uses and sources. Consequently, it is necessary to identify essential data elements that are gathered through a timely and cost-effective process. The topics covered in Part V relate not only to specific analyses but also to key data elements in universal practice.

SUMMARY

Having examined briefly the present hospital environment, the various theories of the causes of the inflation in health care costs, and the components, of the financial cycle, readers must now develop their own thoughts on specific issues and tactics. If there is one universal characteristic of the hospital system, it is that each hospital operates in a unique environment and has adapted to that environment through an adaptive process that provides adequate approaches to financial management. Practices developed over time are now part of the daily routine and are difficult to change. If, in the following sections, new ideas or alternatives can be developed, the result will be well worth the time and effort involved.

To this end, direct involvement with the text material is necessary. Readers who are students (future managers and administrators in the health care field) or practitioners will be, or perhaps already are, confronted with the complex task of directing an institution that delivers care to a dependent service area. As such, the reader's task is to manage resources to achieve goals within specific time frames. There are no fixed answers to many of the questions involved; this will become evident as the many complex issues are presented in the following sections. However, a brief examination of the issues covered thus far may serve to focus the reader's thinking on some key preliminary questions:

- Of the various theories advanced to explain health care inflation, which, in the reader's opinion, are predominant? Discuss the reasons.

- As the new administrator of a 300-bed medical center, the reader is contemplating the possibility of restructuring administrative responsibilities. The present organizational structure is similar to that of Community 1 in Figure 1–1. What changes should be made in the structure? Why?

- Identify the basic components of the financial cycle and describe the necessary interaction between the elements of the cycle.

The case-study approach utilized in the following sections will aid readers in developing their own managerial styles, attitudes, and skills. It is essential to view the case presented as a real hospital that the reader is responsible for. Readers should weigh their evaluations on the assumption that someday, if not already, the facts, theories, frustrations, and achievements presented on these pages will affect them, whatever their organizational positions.

NOTE

1. Van Sewell, *Hospital Accounting—Theory and Practice* (Chicago: Hospital Financial Management Assoc., 1970), pp. 1–25.

Chapter 2

Community Medical Center: The Case Hospital

INTRODUCTION

The position you are to assume in working through this case is that of a new president, the chief executive officer, at Community Medical Center. You have a basic, but very limited knowledge of the center's service area and detailed operations and of the community serviced by the Medical Center. Throughout the case discussion, keep in mind that *you* are responsible for the operations of the facility and the provision of medical care to the population within Community Medical Center's service area. As you proceed, develop a set of questions and observations that you view as critical regarding the institution and its environment and compare these with the facts contained in the presentation.

While the volume of detail in this chapter may appear overwhelming, you should review the data as essential elements in developing opinions regarding the operations and financial position of Community Medical Center. Statistical analyses may be performed on the data, as an interdisciplinary approach to determine significant causal and trend relationships.

Finally, you should understand that Community Medical Center is very interested in a possible expansion of services at this time but that there are limited funds available to finance an expansion project of any magnitude. For this reason, you should be particularly interested in the presentations to be made.

COMMUNITY DEMOGRAPHICS

Community Medical Center is located in the northeastern Illinois community of Steeltown. Steeltown is in Steel County, Illinois, directly across the county line from Chicago. The population of Steeltown is 40,400, based on the 1970 census. The town is a diversified industrial community with convenient access to land, water, and air transportation facilities. Manufacturing forms the basis of the Steeltown economy, accounting for 47 percent of all private, nonfarm income in the county in 1972.

Industries account for 41 percent of the employment in the county, the largest being a steel mill employing about 5,000 people. Median family income in the county in 1969 was $10,249. For Illinois as a whole, the median income was $10,959, and for the United States, $9,586. There are many higher education facilities in the Steeltown area and several fine medical schools in the Chicago area.

THE MEDICAL CENTER

Staffing and Facilities

Community Medical Center is a 350-bed, acute care general hospital. The (licensed) bed complement, based upon service, is as follows:

Medical-surgical	253
Intensive care	12
Pediatric	28
Obstetrics	32
Psychiatric	25
	350

In addition, the center's facilities include a 32-bassinet nursery, six labor rooms, three delivery rooms, a 4-bed obstetrical recovery room, five operating rooms, a 10-bed surgery recovery room, and emergency services staffed by emergency care physicians on a 24-hour per day basis. There are 90 physicians on the medical staff of the center. The specialties and age distribution of these physicians are shown in Table 2–1.

The Community Medical Center was established in 1920 under the governance of the churches in the community. It is a not-for-profit corporation under the rules governing a 501(c)(3) organization. The institution is an area-wide trauma center and is a leader in the provision of services to the area which it serves. Population trends in the center's service area are projected in Table 2–2. The center is the sole provider for the primary service area and serves approximately 85 percent of the area.

Table 2-1 Specialties and Age Distribution of Community Medical
Center Physicians

Specialty	Total
Allergy	2
Cardio-thoracic surgery	3
Dermatology	1
Diagnostic medicine	5
Endocrinology	0
Family practice	15
Gastroenterology	1
Hematology and oncology	0
Nephrology	2
Pediatrics	8
Thoracic medicine	1
General surgery	8
Neurological surgery	1
Obstetrics and gynecology	7
Ophthalmology	3
Oral surgery	5
Orthopedics	2
Otorhinolaryngology	2
Periphro-vascular surgory	1
Plastic surgery	2
Thoracic surgery	0
Urology	2
Anesthesiology	1
Child psychiatry	0
Hyperalimentation	0
Infectious diseases	0
Neurology	1
Pathology	2
Podiatry	0
Psychiatry	6
Radiology	2
Rheumatology	1
Cardiology	6
	90

Age Group	Percent	% of Total Admissions
Under 40	23	22
40–50	31	32
51–60	25	25
Over 60	21	21
	100	100

Table 2-2 Community Medical Center's Service Area: Projected Population Growth—1970/1985

Year	Population	Year	Population
1970	77,025	1978	81,640
1971	77,590	1979	82,240
1972	78,150	1980	82,840
1973	78,720	1981	83,440
1974	79,300	1982	84,050
1975	79,880	1983	84,670
1976	80,460	1984	85,290
1977	81,050	1985	85,910

Occupancy and Services

Community Medical Center provides the customary services offered by a general, acute care facility. These are medical, surgical, obstetrics, pediatrics, intensive care, and psychiatric.

Over the past several years, the center has experienced an increase in the number of identified psychiatric visits. The center projects a continued growth in this area, based on historic trends and as the result of the deinstitutionalizing of mental health patients and the addition of several psychiatrists to the center's staff beginning in 1975. In general, the center is very optimistic about the potential growth in utilization and, based on historical trends, expects the patient-day load to increase in the future.

Ancillary Department Activity

Ancillary department activity at the Community Medical Center has been increasing at a constant pace. As in other general hospitals, ancillary activity accounts for over 50 percent of the gross patient charges, and the percentage reliance on ancillary activity in both inpatient and outpatient areas is increasing annually. At the center, the concentration has been on several key ancillary areas as the focus of increased "marketing" activities.

Laboratory

Since 1973, laboratory tests in both absolute numbers and per admission have increased steadily at the center. The total volume of laboratory activity in both the inpatient and outpatient areas has increased each year. This volume is expected to increase further as the center acquires additional internal capabilities and reduces reliance on outside labs.

Radiology Department

Similarly, in the radiology department there has been a consistent growth in the number of both inpatient and outpatient activities over the past several years. In view of the projected overall growth in inpatient activity, no slow-down in this trend is expected in the near future. A significant fact concerning the number of radiology visits is the high percentage of outpatient activity compared to inpatient services.

At present, the radiology department is in the process of expanding services via specialized procedures made available by technological developments such as the CAT scanner and ultrasound. The medical staff is enthusiastic regarding this equipment, and several internal studies are under way to determine the best locations for future acquisitions.

Emergency Room

A significant entry point for the hospital is through the emergency room (ER). Trauma cases and those patients who do not have a local physician make their initial contact with the hospital through the ER. While the growth in this area has been unsteady, it is felt that the center continues to treat the most serious cases while increases in the medical staff have absorbed the remainder of the illnesses that are better treated in the physician's office. It is believed that increased marketing efforts in the medical staff area could have an impact in attracting those persons who are not treated at the center.

Outpatient Activity

The increased emphasis on cost containment has resulted in a greater awareness that services performed on an outpatient basis are more economical than those performed on persons as inpatients. Outpatient visits and procedures have risen steadily over the past several years and have prompted the center's evaluation of possible expansion in this area. The center is in the process of completing on-site physicians' offices in anticipation of increased utilization by physicians of the center's ancillary services. The on-site offices will also serve as attractive recruitment incentives to add physicians to the center's staff.

Potential Expansion

Community Medical Center is in a position to expand both physically and in service to its service area. At the present growth rate, the center will not have space to meet the increased demands projected above. Increased psychiatric services are reducing the number of medical/surgical beds available, and waiting lists are being created. In the present mobile society, the hospital believes that, in order to retain its market position, it is essential that necessary services be available when needed.

Ancillary services are expanding at such a rate that additional equipment will be necessary in the near future. However, there is no space for the equipment, nor for the personnel required to serve the increased volume of patients. The laboratory and the radiology and emergency rooms are expected to require double the present square footage in the not-too-distant future in order to meet the increasing needs of the patient population. Increasing the square footages in these areas requires additional boiler capacity and supporting services, such as warehouse storage. Increased patient volume requires additional personnel, which will result in the need for increased cafeteria seating and parking.

Therefore, an expansion project has been projected in the following areas: medical records, cafeteria, ancillary areas and storeroom, psychiatric services, and the power plant. The estimated cost of construction is $12 million, and the project would take about three years to complete. The project has been in the planning stages for about nine months, and the center's board is anxious to begin the decision-making process. An architect has been retained by the center to begin rough drawings for further discussions. Illinois has a certificate-of-need law that requires that detailed planning analyses be approved before firm commitments are made regarding construction. The utilization projections are expected to provide the necessary support for the need aspect of the permission application, but the law also requires detailed financial analyses before the application is considered complete. Finally, the local HSA must approve the project as an initial step in the permission application process.

In addition to the proposed construction program, the center is actively involved in marketing and community development programs that emphasize increased utilization through contracting with community agencies and local industries to provide routine services, such as preemployment physicals. There is also some interest in the establishment of shared services between local hospitals, with a view to establishing referral patterns and shared management services.

Finances

Finance in the health care industry is restricted by many environmental pressures. These will put limits on the flexibility required to achieve many of the projects outlined above. Environmental pressures common to all hospitals include cost containment and the possibility of limitations on cost and revenues, restrictions on Medicare and Medicaid reimbursement, dramatic increases in medical malpractice premiums and a resulting growth of self-insurance and risk management programs, and increased scrutiny of hospital operations by the IRS. Moreover, the center has not accumulated sufficient capital to meet the state requirement that not more than 80 percent of the total project cost be covered with borrowed funds. Hill-Burton regulations project changes in the amount of charity funds that can be used for such purposes, designating the specific amounts required per year. Medicare reimbursement principles relate to cost reimbursement only; there is no recognition of bad debts and of certain major operating expenses, such as interest paid during construction. The center's volume of Medicare and Medicaid patients has increased steadily over the past several years, to current levels of 46 percent Medicare and Medicaid and 7 percent Blue Cross, which pays cost plus 5 percent. All of these factors must weigh heavily on the decision-making process for the proposals presented above.

The Community Medical Center has one of the lowest operating costs per patient day in the area and the lowest per-day room charge in the area of private hospitals. Efficiencies must be emphasized, and extreme care must be taken before a major cost, such as that involved in a construction program, is incurred.

Exhibits 2–1 to 2–8 present data from the summary financial statements for Community Medical Center for the years 1977 and 1978. Exhibits 2–9 to 2–16 present corresponding comparative data for the years 1978 and 1979. The statements indicate increased accounts receivable, slight cash accumulation, and provisions for price level depreciation (which is nonreimbursable). Exhibits 2–17 and 2–18 provide inpatient and productivity data for Community Medical Center.

Exhibit 2–1 Community Medical Center: Balance Sheet Assets for the Years 1977 and 1978 Ending December 31

	1978	1977
	(in 000s)	
Current Assets:		
Cash	$ 13	$ 100
Receivables, less reserves for uncollectible accounts and contractual allowances of $995,000 and $885,000	2,941	2,508
Inventories	297	332
Prepaid insurance	31	15
Total current assets	$ 3,282	$ 2,955
Property, Plant, and Equipment, at cost:		
Land	$ 579	$ 503
Land improvements	285	265

Exhibit 2–1 continued

Buildings and building service equipment	16,604	16,545
Departmental equipment	2,979	2,771
Construction in progress	553	28
	$21,000	$20,112
Less accumulated depreciation	7,057	5,938
	$13,943	$14,174
Other Assets:		
Unamortized debt expense	$ 79	$ 96
Board-designated funds for plant expansion: Treasury bills	1,632	1,430
	$ 1,711	$ 1,526
	$18,936	$18,655
Restricted Funds		
Industrial Development Fund:		
Due from unrestricted fund	$ 20	$ —
	$ 20	$ —

Exhibit 2–2 Community Medical Center: Balance Sheet Liabilities and Fund Balances for the Years 1977 and 1978 Ending December 31

	1978	1977
	(in 000s)	
Current Liabilities:		
Current maturities of long-term debt	$ 320	$ 295
Note payable, 12%	10	15
Accounts payable	910	524
Accrued liabilities	595	595
Other reserves	24	18
Due to restricted fund	20	—
Total current liabilities	$ 1,879	$ 1,447
Deferred Revenues, arising from use of accelerated depreciation for Medicare and Medicaid reimbursement	$ 356	$ 340

Exhibit 2-2 continued

Long-Term Debt, less current maturities	$ 5,500	$ 6,000
Fund Balance	$11,201	$10,868
	$18,936	$18,655
Restricted Funds		
Industrial Development Fund: Fund balance	$ 20	$ —
	$ 20	$ —

Exhibit 2-3 Community Medical Center: Statements of Revenues and Expenses, for the Years 1977 and 1978 Ending December 31

	1978	1977
	(in 000s)	
Operating Revenue:		
Gross revenue from patient services:		
Inpatient	$14,513	$12,468
Outpatient	1,458	1,303
	$15,971	$13,771
Revenue deductions	1,510	1,599
Net revenue from patient services	$14,461	$12,172
Other operating revenue	222	179
Total operating revenue	$14,683	$12,351
Operating Expenses:		
Salaries	$ 7,045	$ 5,773
Fees and commissions	1,379	1,193
Supplies	2,748	2,103
Other expenses	1,753	1,178
Interest and amortization of debt expense	520	549
Depreciation-cost	1,125	1,139
Total operating expenses	$14,570	$11,935
Income (loss) from operations	$ 113	$ 416

Exhibit 2-3 continued

Nonoperating Revenue:		
Contributions	21	9
Interest income	143	149
Excess (deficiency) of revenues over expenses	$ 277	$ 574

Exhibit 2-4 Community Medical Center: Statements of Changes in Fund Balances, for the Years 1977 and 1978 Ending December 31

	1978	1977
	(in 000s)	
Unrestricted Funds:		
Balance Beginning of Year	$10,868	$10,157
Add (Deduct):		
Excess (deficiency) of revenues		
over expenses	277	574
Transfer from plant replacement		
fund to finance property and		
equipment additions	56	137
Balance End of Year	$11,201	$10,868
Restricted Funds:		
Industrial Development Fund:		
Balance Beginning of Year	$ —	$ 44
Add (Deduct):		
Grants	—	93
Pledge write-offs	—	(24)
Contributions	76	24
Transfer to unrestricted funds	(56)	(137)
Balance End of Year	$ 20	$ —

Exhibit 2-5 Community Medical Center: Statements of Changes in Financial Position of Unrestricted Funds, for the Years 1977 and 1978 Ending December 31

	1978	1977
	(in 000s)	
Sources of Funds:		
Operations:		
Income (loss) from operations	$ 113	$ 416
Noncash charges against income:		
Provision for depreciation-cost	1,119	1,139
Amortization of debt expense	17	20
Increase in deferred revenues	16	33
Funds provided from operations	1,265	1,608
Contributions and interest income	164	158
Transfer from Industrial Development Fund to finance property and equipment additions	56	137
	$1,485	$1,903
Applications of Funds:		
Additions to property and equipment, net	888	507
Increase in board-designated funds for plant expansion	202	608
Reduction of long-term debt	500	300
	$1,590	$1,415
Increase (Decrease) in Working Capital	$ (105)	$ 488
Changes in Components of Working Capital:		
Current assets, increase (decrease):		
Cash	$ (87)	$ (40)

Exhibit 2–5 continued

Receivables	433	952
Inventories	(35)	50
Prepaid insurance	16	(5)
	$ 327	$ 957
Current liabilities, increase (decrease):		
Current maturities of long-term debt	$ 25	$ 9
Notes payable to banks and other	(5)	(5)
Accounts payable	386	224
Accrued liabilities	—	240
Specific purpose reserve	6	1
Due to restricted fund	20	—
	$ 432	$ 469
Increase (Decrease) in Working Capital	$ (105)	$ 488

Exhibit 2–6 Community Medical Center: Gross Revenue from Patient Services, for the Year 1978 Ending December 31

	(in 000s)		
	Inpatient	Outpatient	Total
General care	$ 5,795	$ —	$ 5,795
Intensive care	487	—	487
Pediatrics	528	—	528
Nursery	116	—	116
Operating room	904	27	931
Recovery room	148	—	148
Delivery room	68	—	68
Anesthesiology	577	15	592
Radiology	855	552	1,407
Nuclear medicine	187	37	224
EEG	76	11	87
Laboratory	1,794	190	1,984
Electrocardiology	352	29	381
Physical therapy	92	81	173

Exhibit 2-6 continued

Pharmacy	1,168	32	1,200
Special procedures	107	15	122
Blood	138	1	139
Medical and surgical	322	15	337
Inhalation therapy	653	5	658
Emergency room	146	448	594
Totals	$14,513	$1,458	$15,971

Exhibit 2-7 Community Medical Center: Other Operating Revenue, for the Year 1978 Ending December 31

	(in 000s)
Cafeteria revenue	$128
Parking lot	28
Recovery of departmental expense	24
Telephone commissions	1
Rental property (loss)	32
Miscellaneous, net	9
Total	$222

Exhibit 2-8 Community Medical Center: Revenue Deductions, for the Year 1978 Ending December 31

	(in 000s)
Allowances:	
Contractual	$ 726
Medical center personnel	35
Charity	82
Other	5
	$ 848
Bad Debts	662
Total	$1,510

Exhibit 2-9 Community Medical Center: Balance Sheet Assets, for the Years 1978 and 1979 Ending December 31

	1979	1978
	(in 000s)	
Current Assets:		
Cash	$ 3	$ 13
Receivables, less reserves for uncollectible accounts and contractual allowances of $824,000 and $995,000	3,273	2,941
Inventories	320	297
Prepaid insurance	32	31
Total current assets	$ 3,628	$ 3,282
Property, Plant, and Equipment, at cost:		
Land	$ 779	$ 579
Land improvements	297	285
Buildings and building service equipment	16,932	16,604
Departmental equipment	3,426	2,979
Construction in progress	1,411	553
	$22,845	$21,000
Less accumulated depreciation	8,126	7,057
	$14,719	$13,943
Other Assets:		
Unamortized debt expense	$ 63	$ 79
Board-designated funds for plant expansion: Certificates of deposit	1,026	1,632
	$ 1,089	$ 1,711
	$19,436	$18,936
Restricted Funds:		
Industrial Development Fund: Due from unrestricted fund	$ —	$ 20

Exhibit 2–10 Community Medical Center: Balance Sheet Liabilities and Fund Balances, for the Years 1978 and 1979 Ending December 31

	1979	1978
	(in 000s)	
Current Liabilities:		
Short Term bank loan, 12%	$ 150	$ —
Current maturities of long-term debt	347	320
Notes payable	95	10
Accounts payable	964	910
Accrued liabilities	674	595
Other reserves	24	24
Due to restricted fund	—	20
Total current liabilities	$ 2,254	$ 1,879
Deferred Revenues, arising from use of accelerated depreciation for Medicare reimbursement	$ 366	$ 356
Long-Term Debt, less current maturities	$ 5,180	$ 5,500
Fund Balance	$11,636	$11,201
	$19,436	$18,936
Restricted Funds:		
Industrial Development Fund: Fund balance	$ —	$ 20

Exhibit 2–11 Community Medical Center: Statements of Revenues and Expenses, for the Years 1978 and 1979 Ending December 31

	1979	1978
	(in 000s)	
Operating Revenue:		
Gross revenue from patient services		
Inpatient	$17,457	$14,513
Outpatient	1,872	1,458
	$19,329	$15,971
Revenue deductions	2,072	1,510
Net revenue from patient services	$17,257	$14,461
Other operating revenue	322	222
Total operating revenue	$17,579	$14,683
Operating Expenses:		
Salaries	$ 8,632	$ 7,045
Fees and commissions	1,793	1,379
Supplies	3,174	2,748
Other expenses	2,088	1,753
Interest and amortization of debt expense	491	520
Depreciation-Cost	1,104	1,125
Total operating expenses	$17,282	$14,570
Income (loss) from operations	$ 297	$ 113
Nonoperating Revenue:		
Contributions	8	21
Interest income	92	143
Excess of revenues over expenses	$ 397	$ 277

Exhibit 2–12 Community Medical Center: Statements of Changes in Fund Balances, for the Years 1978 and 1979 Ending December 31

	1979	1978
	(in 000s)	
Unrestricted Funds:		
Balance Beginning of Year	$11,201	$10,868
Add (Deduct):		
Excess (deficiency) of revenues over expenses	397	277
Transfer from plant replacement fund to finance property and equipment additions	38	56
Balance End of Year	$11,636	$11,201
Restricted Fund:		
Industrial Development Fund:		
Balance Beginning of Year	$ 20	$ —
Add (Deduct):		
Contributions restricted for property and equipment additions	18	76
Transfer to unrestricted funds	(38)	(56)
Balance End of Year	$ —	$ 20

Exhibit 2-13 Community Medical Center: Statements of Changes in Financial Position of Unrestricted Funds for the Years 1978 and 1979 Ending December 31

	1979	1978
	(in 000s)	
Sources of Funds:		
Operations:		
Income from operations	$ 297	$ 113
Noncash charges against income:		
Provisions for depreciation-cost	1,069	1,119
Amortization of debt expense	16	17
Increase in deferred revenues	10	16
Funds provided from operations	$1,392	$1,265
Contributions and interest income	100	164
Transfer from Industrial Development Fund to finance property and equipment additions	38	56
Decrease in board-designated funds for plant expansion	606	—
	$2,136	$1,485
Applications of Funds:		
Additions to property and equipment, net	$1,845	$ 888
Increase in board-designated funds for plant expansion	—	202
Reduction of long-term debt	320	500
	$2,165	$1,590
Increase (Decrease) in Working Capital	$ (29)	$ (105)
Changes in Components of Working Capital:		
Current assets, increase		

Exhibit 2–13 continued

(decrease):		
Cash	$ (10)	$ (87)
Receivables	332	433
Inventories	23	(35)
Prepaid insurance	1	16
	$ 346	$ 327
Current liabilities, increase (decrease):		
Short-term bank loan	$ 150	$ —
Current maturities of long-term debt	27	25
Notes payable	85	(5)
Accounts payable	54	386
Accrued liabilities	79	—
Specific purpose reserve	—	6
Due to restricted fund	(20)	20
	$ 375	$ 432
Increase (Decrease) in Working Capital	$ (29)	$ (105)

Exhibit 2–14 Community Medical Center: Gross Revenue from Patient Services, for the Year 1979 Ending December 31

	Inpatient	Outpatient	Total
		(in 000s)	
General care	$ 7,165	$ —	$ 7,165
Intensive care	617	—	617
Pediatrics	727	—	727
Nursery	161	—	161
Operating room	1,049	30	1,079
Recovery room	180	6	186
Delivery room	73	—	73
Anesthesiology	737	19	756
Radiology	1,196	844	2,040
Nuclear medicine	266	30	296
EEG	85	9	94

Exhibit 2–14 continued

Laboratory	1,797	214	2,011
Electrocardiology	398	35	433
Physical therapy	97	69	166
Pharmacy	1,441	35	1,476
Special procedures	122	13	135
Blood	125	9	134
Medical and surgical	286	18	304
Inhalation therapy	714	6	720
Emergency room	220	535	755
Total	$17,456	$1,872	$19,328

Exhibit 2–15 Community Medical Center: Other Operating Revenue, for the Year 1979 Ending December 31

	(in 000s)
Cafeteria revenue	$178
Parking lot	38
Recovery of departmental expense	34
Telephone commissions	11
Rental property (loss)	42
Miscellaneous, net	19
Total	$322

Exhibit 2–16 Community Medical Center: Revenue Deductions, for the Year 1979 Ending December 31

	(in 000s)
Allowances:	
Contractual	$1,143
Medical center personnel	46
Charity	113
Other	88
	$1,390
Bad Debts	682
Total	$2,072

Exhibit 2–17 Community Medical Center: Inpatient Data

	Admissions	Average Length of Stay	Patient Days
Actual:			
1975	12,000	6.8	83,000
1976	13,000	6.9	90,000
1977	14,000	7.6	109,000
1978	14,500	7.5	108,000
1979	15,000	7.6	114,000
Forecast:			
1980	15,000	7.6	114,000
1981	15,000	7.6	114,000

Exhibit 2-18 Community Medical Center: Selected Productivity Data

	Current Hours (in 000s)	Activity (in 000s)	State	Nation	1978 Estimate	1979 Budget	1977 Actual
General Care:							
R.N.	120		2.19	2.27	1.30	1.43	1.31
L.P.N.	104	83	.72	1.32	1.16	1.25	1.18
Other	240		3.17	2.61	3.41	2.86	3.14
Total	464	83	6.08	6.20	5.87	5.54	5.63
Pediatrics	74	8	8.38	8.00	8.05	8.38	9.64
Special Care Unit	99	14	6.19	7.05	5.14	6.83	5.53
Intensive Care	84	3	17.03	17.77	18.04	21.50	20.56
Respiratory Therapy	52	45	.96	.85	2.26	1.15	1.44
Laboratory	142	755	2.70	2.50	2.08	2.43	2.10
Pharmacy	41	114	.28	.27	.28	.36	.32
Radiology	88	84	1.33	1.30		1.05	1.04
Emergency Room	53	31	1.93	1.61	1.42	1.74	1.51
Man Hours/Pt. Day			17.84	17.42	16.65	17.69	17.49

Part II

The Financial Reporting Function

Having identified the basic hospital environment in Part I, we will now focus our attention on the financial cycle of reporting, action, planning, and control. The first component to be discussed will be that of reporting. Emphasis in this section will be on the accounting process as related to the hospital environment. While a basic understanding of accounting principles is assumed, it is important for the reader to understand key differences in hospital accounting practices and the emphases in the hospital accounting process compared with that of universal, "industrial" accounting.

Chapter 3 defines the hospital accounting process and identifies key accounting issues of particular interest in the hospital field. The accounting process of accumulation and summarization of financial data on an accurate and timely basis will form the framework for this chapter. Internal control theories will be discussed and illustrated via the case of Community Medical Center. Basic guidelines and direction related to the institution's accounting practices must be set at the highest level of the organization so that adequate data are available for input into the decision-making process. The decision-making process is concerned with the sound internal management of fiscal viability and achievement of goals and with the external pressures discussed in Part I, such as cost containment and planning requirements.

One of the most significant factors affecting the hospital industry is that of third party cost reimbursement. Due to the importance of this factor in hospital financial and accounting processes, Chapter 4 is devoted to a summary of cost reimbursement practices. Cost reimbursement has been practiced since the 1950s in Blue Cross reimbursement to hospitals on a "cost plus" basis for inpatient services. However, the focus on cost reimbursement maximization developed with the inception of the Medicare program in 1965. Many of the state-administered Medicaid programs have followed the Medicare program in cost reimbursement, making this a significantly important factor in the hospital industry. It is not unusual for an institution to have over 50 percent of its services provided to cost-reimbursed patients. This volume of activity necessitates the understanding and direct involvement of administrators in the process of cost reimbursement. Settlements are made to a hospital via a cost report prepared at the end of a hospital's fiscal year. Thus, planning activities must be focused to that end. The basics of cost report preparation are illustrated in the case of Community Medical Center.

The accounting for cost reimbursement has a direct impact on a hospital's statement of revenue and expense, examined in Chapter 5. Since only historic costs are reimbursed, revenues based on full charges are reduced by contractual allowances (which represent "lost" net revenue as a result of cost reimbursement). The statement of revenue and expense reflects the results of operations of an institution over a period of time. The operational results reflected in this statement form the basis for a great deal of action planning by the hospital. In order to form opinions adequately to guide future operations of the institution, the administrator must be able to distinguish key issues in the statement. Items such as depreciation methodologies and accrued liabilities must be fully understood in action planning, in maximizing cost reimbursement, and in maintaining a sound financial position. The medical center case study illustrates the significant issues that are directly affected by the highest level of the organization.

While the statement of revenues and expenses relates to the results of operations of the institution, the balance sheet, the subject of Chapter 6, reflects the financial position of the institution. Key issues related to the balance sheet and of increasing importance to the hospital industry include capital available for asset replacement and expansion, the relationship of long-term debt to equity, and the level and change in the balance of accounts receivable. The balance sheet represents key balances and relationships that directly affect the administration's ability to deal with future issues. These issues emerge in the case of Community Medical Center as the proposed expansion program is explored.

The basic summary reports related to the institution's accounting system are the statement of revenues and expenses and the balance sheet. However, from these statements several reports are derived to identify important issues in the financial management of the hospital. Chapter 7 examines several such reports: the statement of change in working capital, the statement of cash flow, and the statement of change in fund balances. The basic data in these reports serve as the foundation for developing other specific reports required by the administration. Again, the medical center case study serves as the vehicle of illustration.

In examining the material in this section, the reader should keep in mind the operations and decisions related to the effective administration of Community Medical Center. As president of the institution, the reader should be prepared to direct operations on the basis of the data presented. Additional data necessary for the formulation of an action plan should be developed from the case presentation and then expanded in the discussions to follow.

Chapter 3

The Hospital Accounting System

INTRODUCTION

In this chapter, in the presentation of the integrated segments of accounting systems, detailed journal entries are provided at various points. In this context, the study and evaluation of accounting forms the basis for auditing practice and as such provides an insight into the assessment of overall accounting practices. This system provides the hospital administration student with a practical overview of and guide to basic accounting.

It should be noted that there are many common accounting objectives among the various segments of the accounting cycle. As a result, the reader may feel that, at some points, the discussion of these objectives is repetitious. However, the elimination of the relevant objectives at such points could be misleading in presenting the evaluation procedures. Thus, for the sake of clarity, these common objectives are cited as necessary at each relevant point in the examination of the segments of the accounting cycle.

The basic objectives of accounting systems is the accumulation, recording, and reporting of financial information on a timely and accurate basis in accordance with "generally accepted accounting principles." While the specific mechanics of accounting operations vary by institution and level of computerization, the basic principles of accounting system design are universal. However, the impact of the type of institution on the accounting system cannot be overestimated. Hospitals are generally voluntary, not-for-profit institutions and as such are exempt from federal income taxes under Section 501(c)(3) of the Internal Revenue Code, which specifies that the hospital be organized as a charitable, nonprofit corporation whose purpose is caring for the sick. No portion of net earnings can benefit any private shareholder or individual. The effects of this type institution on the accounting system design are that income tax liabilities are minimal (only for unrelated business taxable income) and that, generally, all persons desiring services are treated,

43

regardless of ability to pay. Also, private investment capital is minimal, since no one person may benefit from corporate earnings. Receivables accounting and related estimates of revenue deductions are therefore a primary focus of the hospital accounting system. Detailed records must be maintained for each patient seen, and controls must be incorporated into the system for billing, cash receipts, and management reporting. Contributions, which are tax-deductible by the donor, must be accounted for in line with any restrictions placed on the gifts.

In addition, hospitals that are reimbursed under third party cost reimbursement programs must account for contractual allowances, which are the difference between billed charges and the reimbursed costs. Historically, hospitals have followed strict fund accounting principles with separate funds established for operation capital, plant, debt, contributions, and other restricted areas. However, current practices have led to an increased need for clarity in the presentation of financial statements and to a basic redesign of the hospital's financial statements and accounting details. The redesign is outlined in the *Hospital Audit Guide* prepared by the Committee on Health Care Institutions of the American Institute of Certified Public Accountants.[1] The basic philosophy of the redesign is to distinguish clearly funds that are unrestricted from those that are restricted as to operating use. As an example, historically, the hospital building would be classified as part of the plant fund, even though no restrictions had been placed on its use. Presently, this building is a part of the unrestricted assets of the hospital, like land, operating capital, accounts payable, and so on. Restricted funds should be identified only if restrictions exist outside of the normal operations of the hospital. The financial statements for Community Medical Center reflect the principles outlined in the *Hospital Audit Guide* and should be reviewed at this time by the reader (see Chapter 2).

THE ACCOUNTING FUNCTION

As previously noted, the accounting function has several basic objectives keyed to the various components of the financial cycle. The data accumulation function is crucial in all of the components. Any transaction affecting the finances of the institution must be incorporated into the accounting system for processing. The information must be collected in a format that is applicable to accounting summarization. Each event must be analyzed to determine whether there is an effect on the accounting process and to determine the proper disposition of the information pertinent to the finances of the institution. The basic procedures of data accumulation are summarized in Figure 3–1.

Source documents are the entry points for data into the accounting system. In order to ensure a systematic flow of work through the system, several key elements of systems design must be considered.

- *Centralization.* There must be a central location designed for the document flow into the accounting system. At this point, checks and balances of the main functions are appropriate.

- *Documentation.* Documents must contain all information pertinent to the analysis and recording of the transaction. No transaction is valid unless full documentation is obtained.

- *Authorization.* There must be identifiable authorization and follow-up responsibility for the transaction related to the document.

- *Document control.* Control must be imposed on the documents to avoid loss or duplication of processing. Separation of this control from the controller's office is advisable.

- *Collection.* Systems of data collection must be developed to effect the systematic and timely flow of data into the accounting system.

- *Control.* Control verification must be performed on the documents to ensure the accuracy of information contained in the documentation of the transaction. Accountability for this should be to the hospital's board.

The above elements are the responsibility of the administration of the hospital and must be thoroughly understood to eliminate the possibility of misunderstanding. All procedures must be documented and communicated to all affected areas of the institution.

Financial data originate at various locations of the institution. System objectives are designed to capture these data to achieve timely, accurate, and cost-effective data collection for the accounting system. The following basic accounting functions or cycles may be used to isolate key areas for identification of central location and work flow.

Cash Control Cycle

The cash control cycle is concerned with the institution's capital funds, which include cash, investments, debt management, and various restricted fund balances. Most of the functions performed in the cash control cycle are performed at the treasurer or controller level in the organization, but other areas, such as employee benefits, may also be involved. Transactions common to the cash control cycle include investment of cash, that is, the

Figure 3–1 Accounting Data Flow

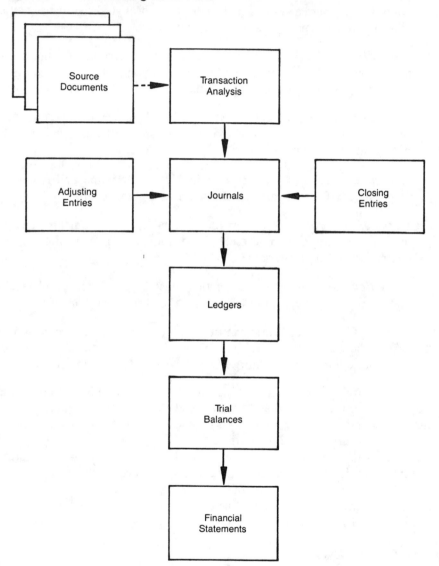

purchase and sale of investment instruments; issuance of both short- and long-term debt; payments of principal and interest to service the debt; deposits and withdrawals from checking accounts; management of pension funds; and management of self-insurance trusts and other liquid assets held in trusts.

Due to the liquidity of cash and investments, it is imperative that centralization be maintained for these transactions at the highest organizational levels and that detailed authorization procedures be established. Only a small number of persons in the organization should be authorized and made responsible by the board of directors for initiating transactions associated with this cycle. It is not uncommon for the board to place restrictions on transactions capable of being performed by a single individual in the organization. For example, the controller alone may be authorized to write checks for up to $100,000, but higher amounts may require the authorization of two or more persons, say the controller and a vice-president; higher amounts may require board approval, depending on the size of the hospital. All checking, savings, investment, and trusteed accounts must be approved by the institution's board to ensure direct involvement at the highest possible level, thereby strengthening corporate control of the liquid assets of the institution. The purpose and location of these accounts must be approved by the board.

In the development of an accounting system to deal with the transactions of the cash control cycle, one must keep in mind the six points of document control previously discussed.

Centralization

While various authorizations for transactions may be required, there must be a central location within the organization where all transactions are coordinated. The need for this centralization is readily apparent in the case of transactions in the cash control cycle. For example, if the controller and president are authorized to issue checks, there is the possibility that without centralization duplicate checks may be prepared or bank overdrafts will be created by the volume of checks issued by each person. Generally, centralization is coordinated at the highest possible level in the finance area of the organization, usually by the vice-president of finance or the controller, with continued safeguards for separate duties.

Documentation

There are many types of documents related to the cash control cycle:

- initial authorization for the transaction
- transaction documentation in accordance with board requirements

- external verification by bank, trustee, or investment banker to an independent party
- safekeeping of documents purchased or sold
- periodic reports to the board of balances and transactions, such as bank statements and investment statements

The initial authorization for a transaction affecting the cash control cycle must include a date, description of the transaction, amount of the transaction, and authorization, usually in the form of the signatures of those persons authorized to initiate the transaction. Formats for authorization vary from internal memos to preprinted forms; the format generally is not as important as the information contained in the authorization document.

Authorization

In addition to identifying the persons authorized to initiate transactions, it is important to identify those persons authorized to carry out the authorized transactions. For example, the controller may authorize the issuance of a check, but the actual writing and disbursement of the check may be done by an accountant in the accounting department. Specific procedures must be identified and agreed to by top management regarding the implementation of authorized transactions. Each transaction document must identify the disposition and classification of the authorized event; for this purpose, written procedures are necessary.

Document Control

Once the transaction is authorized, documents must be centralized and controlled in order to provide resource documentation of the transaction, support for the transaction, and assurance that the documents will not be lost or used again in an effort to obtain unauthorized funds. In addition to the authorization and transaction documents, verification documents from the outside institution for the transaction should be controlled with the internal documents so that a complete documentation of the transaction can be maintained for future reference. In the case of investments or funds held by a trustee, verification of the documents held in safekeeping accounts by the outside institution should be controlled by a person outside of the initial authorization process. Source documents such as stock certificates and bonds should be held in a safe or safety deposit box, with access restricted to only two independent and authorized parties.

External confirmations of transactions must be analyzed by an independent person from either the authorizing or record keeping agents. External confirmations include bank statements, vendor statements of account, investment statements, and periodic reports from trustees. Each analysis should verify balances reported by the institution and identify any interfund transfers. At this point, source documents should be analyzed for completeness and discrepancies should be reported to top management. The analysis should be reported in detail to the board.

Collection of Data

The accounting system must provide for complete and timely collection of data and documents to enable the reporting function to provide the most current information for managerial decision making. The centralization of data accumulation significantly reduces the possibility of time delays and incomplete documentation, but care must be taken to ensure that no outstanding transactions exist after a reporting period is ended. Such "cut-off" problems may result in material misstatement of the operations and position of the institution. As an example, consider the following case. On April 30, $500,000 is received in interest on a particular investment. If this is not recorded on a timely basis, revenue and cash balances will be understated by $500,000. This significant misstatement could result in important alterations in management decision making. By simply reviewing received documents for a short time after the end of the fiscal period and performing a reconciliation of external verification, the chance of such problems arising may be reduced substantially. In short, periodic, independent review is essential.

Internal Control

As noted earlier, control considerations are inherent in the functions of authorization, verification of external documents, and centralization. The control issues in the cash control cycle can be described in terms of the following key objectives.

Authorization objectives should require the following:

- All sources of capital funds, that is, debt, contributions, payables, and so forth, should be authorized in accordance with criteria approved by top management and the board in writing.

- The amounts, timing, and conditions of debt transactions should be authorized in line with management's criteria.

- Investments must be authorized via criteria established by top management; responsibility and accountability in this area are crucial.

- Detailed procedures should be approved by top management, then written and communicated to those responsible for the various sections of the cash control cycle.

Transaction objectives should cover the following requirements:

- Only those authorized to initiate transactions should be allowed to do so.
- Only those transactions that are in line with management's criteria should be allowed.
- All transactions should be properly reported on a timely basis.
- Interest income, gains, and losses on transactions in the cash control cycle, including changes in market values, should be reported fully and on a timely basis.
- Separation of duties must be maintained, that is, those persons responsible for authorization should be separate from those who perform recording, and independent reconciliation and verification functions should be maintained; separation of duties may be maintained not only by procedure but also by physical and organizational position.

Classification objectives should require the following:

- Journal entries for amounts related to the cash control cycle should be prepared for each transaction and for each accounting period and should be maintained as a function separate from the transaction itself.
- Summary reports should be prepared in accordance with the criteria established by top management.
- Care must be taken to eliminate cut-off errors at the end of the reporting cycle.

Physical safeguard objectives should include the following requirements:

- Access to cash and securities should be permitted only in accordance with top management procedures.
- Access to records should be restricted to authorized personnel.

The above basic criteria and objectives apply to all functions in the accounting cycle. From this perspective, the reader should begin to see not only the detailed accounting criteria that are involved but also the vast amount of administration input and responsibility required in the design and operation of the accounting and finance functions.

Purchasing Expenditure Cycle

The purchasing expenditure cycle relates to the functions involved in the acquisition of supplies from outside vendors. Direct interface with the cash control cycle is made through the accounts payable functions from which payments are made for goods and services. Economic objectives, such as obtaining the best goods and services at the least possible cost, must constantly guide the operations of the purchasing expenditure cycle.

Throughout the cycle, authorization objectives should include the following requirements:

- Top management must develop criteria for vendor approval and authorization. Quality, need, and price are key factors related to vendor selection. Bid lists are essential.
- Only authorized persons should be allowed to place orders, and the types, estimated quantities, prices, and terms of goods and services should be authorized only in accordance with management criteria. All purchases must be made via purchase orders.
- Expenditures should be made only in accordance with approval procedures and documentation required by the cash control cycle. The transaction documents transmitted to the cash control cycle must accord fully with the system's objectives described earlier.

Transaction processing objectives should contain the following elements:

- Centralization of the operations of the purchasing function should be maintained. All orders should be placed by the purchasing department at the authorized request of hospital department areas. This centralization is essential for the control of orders in accordance with management criteria, the establishment of economic orders, and the maintenance of efficient data processing. In this context, administrative, budget, and board approval may be required.
- Orders should be made only by approved purchase orders signed by an authorized agent of the hospital and based on bids and administrative approval.
- Only those goods and services requested by the hospital in accordance with approved procedures should be accepted by the receiving area.
- Documentary evidence of the order, receipt, and invoice should be centrally located in the accounting department as authorization for payment.
- Goods and services accepted should be accurately and promptly reported. Resulting vendor liabilities should be promptly verified and reported. Invoices should be sent to an area other than receiving.
- Payments should be made only for authorized liabilities and should be promptly reported as a reduction of the liability incurred.
- The purchasing function should be independent of the recording, payment, and receiving functions.

- Receiving department procedures should require a physical count and verification of items received. Also, the ordering department, purchasing agent, and accounting department should be notified by the receiving department of the receipt of goods or the performance of services.

Classification objectives should encompass the following requirements:

- Data pertaining to a verifiable liability must be recorded via journal entry on a timely basis after the receipt of the goods or services and the incurrence of the liability. The recording must be separate from the purchasing and receiving functions.
- Proper classification of the goods or services must be made based on the type and area of the benefit of the goods or services. That is, the ordering area, including the proper accounting classification, for example, supplies, fees, repairs, and so on—should be identifiable from the data related to the order. No payments are made unless the documentation is complete.
- All entries must be recorded on a timely and accurate basis.

Physical control objectives should include the following requirements:

- All documents pertaining to vendors, payables, and receiving can be accessed only by authorized personnel of the institution. The number of authorized persons must be reduced to the lowest possible number in order to maintain adequate control and accountability. This avoids confidential data being accessed by other vendors.
- Authorization documents for payment and ordering must be voided after use so that no duplication can occur.
- Access to inventory and storage must be restricted.

Payroll Expenditure Cycle

Salary expenses account for about 60 percent of the average hospital's operating expenses. For this reason, close managerial controls are essential to the payroll area. The vast amount of data involved in the personnel function requires systematic accounting procedures in this area. Managerial accounting information flows must be geared not only to internal functions but also to compliance with external controls and requirements, such as federal, state, and local income taxes, unemployment compensation reports, pension reports, federal wage and hour laws, and Social Security (F.I.C.A.) taxes. Accuracy, efficiency, flexibility, and timeliness are essential to the design of the payroll expenditure cycle.

Authorization objectives in the payroll expenditure cycle should include the following requirements:

- Employees should be hired in accordance with procedures established by the hospital's administration and board. Procedures involving direct administrative input include criteria for adding needed personnel, approval procedures for filling vacancies, and controls on the addition of temporary personnel and the expansion of hours of part-time employees.

- Overall and specific wage rates must be approved at the administrative level, and authorization must be obtained before the establishment or alteration of wage rates.

- Employee authorization must be obtained for payroll deductions and levels of withholding for federal, state, and local income taxes requiring W–4 and W–5 forms.

- Supervisor authorization for payment must be obtained via time cards and authorized forms before the payroll area can process data for payment.

Transaction processing objectives should include the following elements:

- The personnel department must be the central location for processing additions to and deletions of staff. All personnel functions must be handled in this central area.

- The payroll department must be the central location for the processing of documents and data required to issue payroll checks.

- Documents flowing into the payroll system, including time records, withholding documents, and classification and wage rates, must be clear, precise, and submitted on a timely and accurate basis.

- Control documents for each employee must be accurate and must contain the data necessary for all required reporting. All salary and hour amounts and individual deductions reports must be cumulative. All control documents must be in a format that facilitates report preparation.

- Detailed and summary reports must be directed to the cash control cycle for payment. Summary reports must flow to the accounting area for timely recording and reporting.

- Distribution functions must be segregated from the data accumulation process and cash control cycle. Paychecks must be distributed only to individual employees, and controls must be maintained to ensure that no checks are lost or stolen.

• Amounts due to or on behalf of employees should be recognized as liabilities on a timely basis. These include accrued wages and taxes, withholdings from employees, and earned, vested vacation pay.

• Verification of payroll and personnel activities must be made on a periodic basis. This should include actually seeing the employees paid.

Classification objectives should include the following requirements:

• Payroll disbursements, related adjustments, and journal entries for amounts due to or on behalf of employees should be prepared for each accounting period. This should be done in an area separate from payroll.

• Entries must be maintained for salaries incurred in the service area of the hospital.

Finally, physical safeguard objectives must require that access to personnel records, payroll records, and checks is restricted to authorized personnel only. Emphasis on control here is crucial, due to the sensitive and confidential nature of the data.

Revenue Cycle

The hospital revenue cycle is the cycle in which it is most critical and difficult to control financial functions. As previously noted, the general hospital must provide service to all who request it, regardless of the ability to pay. Also, the vast number of people insured by a large number of insurance companies requires that the service be performed, coverage information obtained and verified, and a billing cycle maintained for all persons treated at the hospital. Credit policies must be under close administrative supervision and control to ensure adherence to the financial and philosophical objectives of the institution. The volume of services performed by the hospital complicates the data flow in the revenue cycle. It is not uncommon for daily charge entries to total 5,000 items. Thus, controls must be placed on charge creation and alteration as well as on charge collection.

Authorization objectives should require that authorization and documentation are obtained from several sources in the revenue cycle. Authorization for treatments to be performed must be obtained initially from patients at the entry points of the hospital. Consent-to-admit forms are commonly used for this purpose. Also, forms for the assignment of insurance benefits must be signed by the patient to enable the hospital to bill on the patient's behalf and to receive payment directly from the insurance company. The administration of the hospital is responsible for the establishment of admission policies, treatment criteria, and credit policies regarding patient and hospital responsibilities for payment. All services performed by the hospital must be ordered and authorized by the patient's physician or the physician agent of the attending physician. All charges must be authorized by the administration, and billings for service must be authorized by a designated hospital agent. Specifically, the following control points are required:

- Criteria for patient admission and services must be adhered to in authorizing patients to enter the hospital for treatment.
- Authorization for services, prices, and credit must be obtained and adhered to.
- All adjustments to accounts receivables and write-offs of accounts as uncollectable must be authorized in accordance with administrative criteria.
- Revenue cycle processing procedures should be authorized by the administration and should be adhered to throughout the processing phase.

Transaction processing objectives should include the following requirements:

- All data must be centralized and individualized for patients. This centralization is usually the responsibility of the hospital's business office, which holds all data on each patient that are pertinent to the revenue cycle.
- All insurance information, including assignments of benefits, must be collected at points of entry to the hospital, usually the emergency room and the inpatient/outpatient admitting office. The collected information must be transferred intact to the business office for inclusion in the patient's data folder.
- Charge items must be identified, and authorized charges must be controlled by the hospital's administrative personnel, usually by the controller. Unit charges must be given to the business office for charge reference and processing.
- Data on all unit services performed for each patient must be ordered by the physician on the patient areas and transmitted to the business office for charging in accordance with the authorized charge structure. The order must flow to the ancillary area responsible for carrying out the order.
- Billing procedures must be completed as soon as possible after the completion of services. All necessary data must be sent to the business office on a frequent and timely basis for billing completion.

- Credit policies must be adhered to regarding the use of collection agencies and bank arrangements, and approval procedures for charge adjustments must be adhered to.
- Accountability for cash receipts should be established for direct input into the cash control cycle.
- Billed and performed services must be accurately posted to service areas that perform the ordered function. Such postings and periodic billings to patients and insurers must be made on a timely basis.
- Verification of account balances should be performed on a periodic basis. This verification can be handled via periodic billings to patients and confirmation of balances sent out by independent parties.

Classification objectives should require the following:

- Journal entries should be prepared for each transaction in the revenue cycle for each accounting period.
- Revenue journal entries should summarize and classify economic activities in accordance with criteria established by the administration.

Physical safeguard objectives should cover the following requirements:

- Access to cash receipts must be restricted to authorized personnel, and such receipts must be transferred intact to the cash control cycle in accordance with management's criteria.
- Access to patient folders, charge tickets, and adjustment input devices must be restricted to persons authorized by administration.

The vast volume of data and the speed and accuracy of processing required in the revenue cycle lend themselves to computerization and mechanical data processing. Probably the most common systems design in the patient billing cycle is that of data collection via cathode ray tube in each ancillary area and on each patient floor. Orders are entered by patient number on the floors, the orders are sent to the ancillary area, and the order is charged for at the time of order in the business office. While this procedure is faster and more accurate than manual systems, the same processing objectives listed above apply.

Although our discussion has been limited to patient service portions of the revenue cycle, hospitals receive an increasing amount of revenues from other sources, for example, the cafeteria, parking, rentals, and contributions. The same systems objectives noted above must be adhered to in the processing of data and cash from these other sources of revenue.

Asset Expenditure Cycle

As expenditures are made, they may be classified either as current expenses or as deferred expenses to be consumed in the future (assets). Assets that are to be consumed in future periods must be allocated to the period in which they are used. Generally, inventories, prepaid expenses, and capital assets require the use of control objectives in the conversion of an asset into an expense. The control points to be observed as objectives in the development of accounting systems in the asset expenditure cycle are illustrated in the following paragraphs.

Authorization objectives should require the following control points:

- Capital acquisitions, levels of amounts to be capitalized, inventory levels, and levels of prepayment should be authorized only in accordance with top management's criteria.

- Direct administrative authorization must be adhered to for the methods and periods of the amortization of deferred costs, for example, depreciation methods and asset lives. Board input here is essential.

- Property dispositions are made only with administration's authorized criteria. Bids should be open and not secret.

- Inventory procedures, adjustments to inventory levels, property adjustments, and adjustments to levels of other deferred charges should be made in accordance with administrative criteria.

Transaction processing objectives should include the following requirements:

- Only those assets authorized by management are acquired through the purchasing expenditure cycle.

- Once the assets are acquired, specific criteria must be followed regarding the appropriate amortization process. For example, inventory systems provide for periodic or perpetual identification of inventory levels, last-in-first-out (LIFO) or first-in-first-out (FIFO) methods. Capital systems provide for straight-line and accelerated methods of depreciation. Prepaid expenses may be allocated with methods of depreciation on an actual or estimated periodic basis.

- Resources must be accurately and promptly reported, and dispositions and amortization levels must be reported on an accurate and timely basis.

Classification objectives should require the following:

- Journal entries should be prepared for each accounting period for all elements of the asset expenditure cycle.
- Asset expenditure details should be prepared and verified for completeness and accuracy.
- Periodic verification is essential to ensure that reported levels are accurately computed and summarized.

Finally, physical safeguard objectives should require that access to inventory, capital assets, and related documents is restricted to authorized personnel only.

Summary

Key elements of the cycles in the hospital's accounting systems may be summarized as follows:

- Authorization of systems design rests with the hospital's board of directors and the hospital administration.
- Data collection areas and processing areas must be centralized in as few areas as specialization will allow.
- Duties related to authorization, data and cash collection, and reporting must be segregated.
- The systems must allow for full documentation and information flow on an accurate and timely basis.
- Control of documents must be maintained to avoid lost or duplicate transactions.

THE FINANCIAL RECORDING FUNCTION

An understanding of financial recording functions in the hospital requires an identification of the basic reports and procedures necessary to capture and record data for detailed and summarized use. The general accounting principles related to the recording functions may be summarized by the formula

$$Assets = Liabilities + Fund\ Balances$$

Journal entries are based on double entry bookkeeping procedures in which assets have debit balances and both liabilities and fund balances have credit balances. Consequently, increases in assets are debit entries, increases in liabilities are credit entries, and increases in fund balances are credit entries. Each journal entry must have all debits equal to all credits.

The organizational format of hospital recording is the chart of accounts. This lists account numbers and associated account descriptions used in preparing journal entries. The basic outline of hospital recording is the *Chart of Accounts for Hospitals.*[2]

In this chart of accounts, asset accounts are numbered in the 1000 series. Liability and equity accounts are numbered 2000 to 2199 for liabilities and 2200 through 2299 for equity/fund balance accounts. The 3000 series is for revenues from nursing services, the 4000 series is for other professional services, and 5000 through 5499 are for other operating revenues. The numbers 5500 through 5999 are for deductions from revenue. The 6000 series is for nursing service expenses, the 7000 for other professional service expense, the 8000 series for other and general service expense, and the 9000 series for nonoperating revenues. This design is suggestive only; each hospital is free to revise the chart for the desired level of detail required by managerial objectives.

Each cycle outlined in the previous section has subsidiary ledgers for the recording of detailed financial information in line with the requirements of the cycle. A sample listing of subsidiary ledgers for each cycle is shown in Table 3–1.

Table 3–1 Subsidiary Ledgers for Recording Financial Data by Cycle

Cash Control Cycle:

    1. Investment transactions by type
    2. Debt service schedule
    3. Check registers
    4. Accounts payable registers
    5. Restricted fund detail for endowments

Purchasing Cycle:

    1. Vendor lists and bids
    2. Purchase orders
    3. Vendor activity

Payroll Cycle:

    1. Individual earnings
    2. Departmental wages and hours
    3. Benefit accruals by employee

Table 3-1 continued

Revenue Cycle:

1. Account receivable trial balances
2. Carrier trial balances
3. Cash receipts
4. Charge journals
5. Departmental posting journals of charges

Control Cycle:

1. Detailed property records
2. Inventory activity
3. Periodic physical inventories
4. Prepaid expense detail

Each entry in the detailed journals is transmitted to the accounting area for further processing. In the accounting department, journal entries are prepared for the data supplied from the various cycles and are entered into the general journal, which is the accumulation point for all journal entries. Each entry must have the date, account number, account description, debit and credit amounts, a unique identification code, and reference to source documents and/or authorization of entries in the detail journals.

The accounts in the chart of accounts constitute the hospital's trial balance, and the sum of accounts is the general ledger for the hospital. The trial balance lists accounts and balances, while the general ledger gives the detail of journal entries posted to that account as referenced from the general journal. Journal entries are posted to the general ledger of each account where reference numbers, dates, and debit or credit amounts are posted. A summary listing of the general ledger accounts forms the trial balance. At the end of the accounting period, adjusting journal entries are prepared to correct any misclassifications in the accounts, and closing entries are prepared to transfer all revenue and expense amounts to the fund balance account.

THE REPORTING FUNCTION

The recording of transaction data in the formats described above has as its basic objective the reporting of the results of financial operations and the financial position of the hospital via financial statements prepared in accordance with generally accepted accounting principles. The following criteria govern the preparation of financial statements:

- The information contained in the financial statements must be relevant to the users of the financial statements and to the making of economic decisions.

- The data must be understandable to the user.

- The information must be verifiable, based on fact, not assumptions or unreasonable estimations.

- The information must be reported on a timely basis so that decisions and evaluations can be made in a relevant action time frame.

- The financial statements for various periods must be comparable and consistent in preparation. Trend evaluations and analyses depend on comparisons of like elements of data.

- The financial statements must be complete and disclose significant data of value in the evaluation of the institution.

At this point, the reader should review the financial statements of Community Medical Center for 1978 as presented in Chapter 2. The center's statement of revenue and expense, balance sheet, statement of change in fund balance, and statement of change in working capital should be evaluated to determine compliance with the above statements of objectives. Remember that the notes to these financial statements (not shown in the statements of our case study hospital) would be important in the presentation of supporting information in fulfillment of disclosure requirements.

In the financial reporting function, the hospital administrator must constantly evaluate the adequacy of data presented for decision-making inputs. It is essential that interim financial statements be compared with projected financial data as a basis for continually evaluating current positions and the results of actions in the light of planning objectives. Effective corrective action can be taken as necessary only if data are received on a timely basis. Compliance with cycle objectives must be evaluated continuously, and corrective action must be taken to ensure that established procedures are followed. When, as often happens, the financial data are inadequate for decision making, statistical data must be incorporated into the financial cycle and summarized at the discretion of the administration to ensure that key levels of activity, for example, patient days and internal activity levels such as man hours, are taken into account in the decision-making process.

COMMUNITY MEDICAL CENTER

Evaluation of the Purchasing Expenditure Cycle

As president of Community Medical Center, the reader should be keenly aware of the need for full administrative involvement in and understanding of the financial cycle's systems and results. At this point, the reader should begin an evaluation of the existing systems at Community Medical Center by analyzing the center's purchasing expenditure cycle. As a basis for this, the reader should reexamine the basic structure of the accounting area and the organizational positions of those involved in the purchasing cycle (see Figure 3–2 and organizational data in Chapter 2).

Figure 3–2 Community Medical Center: Accounting Department Organization Chart

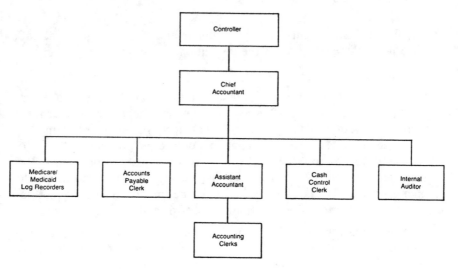

Purchasing

Purchasing for the medical center is done by a purchasing manager. This person purchases for all departments except pharmacy. The pharmacy does its own ordering and receiving, for which invoices are sent directly to purchasing where they are approved and sent to the accounts payable clerk. Dietary is supplied by an outside service, which also runs the food services. The hospital pays for dietary services. Maintenance does part of its own purchasing but must get a purchase order from the purchasing department. The purchasing functions are separate from those of accounting, receiving, and inventory control.

Purchases are made only on the basis of purchase requisitions signed by a department head. When capital items in excess of $150 are requested, they are also approved by a member of the administrative team. When the requisition is for items that have not been ordered before and is in excess of $100, competitive bids must be obtained if possible from at least three vendors. The lowest-bid vendor or the vendor who is most efficient, considering price, delivery time, and service based on the purchasing manager's decision, is selected. If items are reorders, the usual vendor is selected. A five-part, prenumbered purchase order is prepared showing quantities, terms, prices, and the ordering department. The receiving copy is complete as to quantity and description. The copies of the purchase order are distributed as follows: (1) vendor, (2) purchasing, (3) ordering department, (4) receiving (used as a receiving report), and (5) accounts payable. Purchase orders are prenumbered and are filed numerically by the purchasing department. A copy of any voided purchase order is also filed numerically.

The purchasing department, accounting, and the controller's office maintain a list of vendors from whom purchases are made. The list is reviewed periodically by individuals in each of these areas. Each month, the purchasing manager submits a purchasing savings report and a new product evaluation and price report to the administration.

The purchasing manager tries to order in the most economical quantities, taking into consideration use and storage space. The purchasing manager informs the department head who ordered the material of discounts for lot purchases. The department head determines whether large quantities are to be ordered. For purchase order changes, a notice of purchase order change is prepared, and the same distribution is made as for the purchase order. In the case of goods returned, a returned goods requisition is given to the purchasing manager, who contacts the vendor and arranges for the return.

Invoices are never handled by the purchasing department, except where errors have been discovered by accounts payable. Errors may involve higher cost, lower cost, and so forth. The purchasing department will contact the supplier and change the center's price list as needed.

The center gives the purchasing department a budget-approved list of items to be purchased during the year. This list is only for capital items. The purchasing manager does not need approval to purchase items under $500. Approval on a per item basis is needed from administration for items over $500. For medical supplies, solutions, and sutures that are recurring purchases from the same vendors throughout the year, competitive bids must be obtained at the beginning of the year.

Receiving

The receiving department receives all material for all departments except pharmacy and dietary, which receive direct. The receiving department counts all items received, signs and dates the receiving copy of the purchase order, and sends it to accounts payable. For short shipments, the receiving department sends the packing slip to accounts payable for payment in order to obtain the time discounts granted by vendors for prompt payment. The receiving copy of the purchase order is sent to accounts payable only when the order is complete. The receiving department delivers all items to the departments ordering them and gets a department signature showing that the items were received. This is also done for partial shipments. The receiving department sends the receiving copy of the purchase order to accounts payable only when the shipment is complete, except in the case of standby orders where a copy of the purchase order is made and given to accounts payable showing that the portion of the order has been completed. On orders where the quantity received is only a few items short or over the quantity ordered, the merchandise received will be accepted if the department head authorizes it by signing the receiving report and by marking the report "OK" to receive.

Accounts Payable

The hospital maintains an open invoice file. All bills are paid monthly on the tenth of the month or whenever payment is required to enable the hospital to take available discounts. In order to take full advantage of discounts, the hospital maintains a list of vendors who allow discounts even when the terms are not on the invoice. When possible, checks are prepared by a computerized service bureau. On rush items where the discount will be lost if delayed payments are made, a manual check is prepared. Manual checks account for about 30 percent of the checks written.

The accounts payable clerk receives all vendor invoices. The invoices are sent to the assistant controller for approval of payment and periodically to the administrative team. The invoice is matched to the purchase order and receiving reports for payment. The matching process by the accounts payable clerk takes place prior to the payment approval. After the invoices are approved for payment, they are given to the chief accountant who determines the account distributions and fills out the forms for key punching into the computer for the preparation of checks. The chief accountant batches the invoices and prepares batch totals (account numbers and net amount of checks to be processed in the batch) before sending the data to the key punch center located in the business office. The chief accountant fills out a batch control slip for each batch given to the key punch center.

The keypuncher then key punches the batches and inputs the batches into the system to verify the batch totals. Verification of the computed batch totals from the system is given to the chief accountant. Errors are corrected only by the chief accountant. The chief accountant also determines when checks are to be processed. Normally this is done when items are normally processed at the tenth of the month. The system is given the authorization to print checks, which are delivered sealed the following day to the chief accountant.

To note discrepancies, checks are matched against the invoices to be paid. The chief accountant then runs the checks through the check signer. The checks are then given to the accounts payable clerk for mailing. The check copy, paid invoice, purchase orders, receiving report, and other documents are all marked "paid" by the accounts payable clerk and are filed by the name of the vendor.

If a revision of the vendor listing is needed, the chief accountant fills out an accounts payable vendor add-revise-or-delete form for key punching. This is used to update for changes in the vendor listing.

At the end-of-the-month processing, the chief accountant requests a printout of the month's activity by account distribution. An accounts payable release authorization form is used for this purpose. From this listing, the general ledger is posted to the various expense accounts.

Clerical Tests

All invoices are checked when received by the accounts payable clerk. Also, both the assistant controller, when approving the invoices for payment, and the chief accountant, when preparing the account distribution, scan the invoices for reasonableness.

When manual checks are prepared, the invoices go through the same approval process as for checks prepared by the automation system. After approvals are obtained, the checks are typed by the assistant accountant and given back to the chief accountant for signing. A check protector is used for these checks. The checks are mailed to the vendors or are distributed to those who have requested and been approved for receipt of such checks. Manual checks are requested through disbursement vouchers. Approval for the manual checks must come from the controller, president, executive vice-president, or vice-president.

The President's Evaluation

The reader has now been introduced to the purchasing expenditure cycle of Community Medical Center and has also evaluated the various aspects of effective systems design. At this point, the reader should be able to:

* prepare a flow chart of the purchasing expenditure cycle for Community Medical Center, and
* evaluate and compare the center's system with that presented in this chapter. The reader should point out any weaknesses and redesign the system to meet the reader's specifications.

NOTES

1. American Institute of Certified Public Accountants, *Hospital Audit Guide* (New York: American Institute of Certified Public Accountants, 1972).
2. American Hospital Association, *Chart of Accounts for Hospitals* (Chicago: American Hospital Association, 1976).

Chapter 4

Cost Reimbursement under Medicare

INTRODUCTION

Before discussing in detail the significant areas of hospital accounting, an analysis of Medicare principles is essential. The present chapter provides an overview of Medicare principles and practices, the development of Medicare, the effects of Medicare, and the potential future of the Medicare program. The factual exposition of general Medicare practices presented here is followed by an indepth analysis of Medicare management later in the book.

In general, the Medicare program reimburses hospitals on a reasonable, historic cost basis for only those costs related to the care of a covered Medicare patient. Only bad debts related to the Medicare patient's deductible and coinsurance (the portion of the bill for covered services that is not paid by Medicare) are reimbursable. Other bad debts and charity allowances that are incurred through normal hospital operations are not reimbursable. The key to hospital cost reimbursement under Medicare is the determination of the reasonable costs of providing services and the allocation of those costs to the services provided to Medicare beneficiaries. The general procedures related to cost finding and reporting will be discussed later in this chapter. Here it may be noted that the Medicare program accounts for a significant proportion of the revenue of the hospital. This fact has led to serious concern over the ability of the hospital to survive under strict cost reimbursement without regard to current levels of inflation and to the need to earn a return on investment that will provide for asset replacement and improvements. (Medicare does recognize such a return for for-profit hospitals.)

DESCRIPTION AND DEFINITIONS

Medicare—Title XVIII, Health Insurance for the Aged, of the Social Security Act—is a nationwide health insurance program for people aged 65 and over, for persons eligible for social security disability payments for over two years, and for certain workers and their dependents who need kidney transplantation or dialysis.[1] Medicare is financed by payroll taxes on employers and employees and by monthly premiums paid by beneficiaries, all of which is put into special trust funds.[2]

Medicare consists of two separate programs: hospital insurance (Part A) and supplementary medical insurance (Part B). The hospital insurance program is the compulsory portion of Medicare that automatically enrolls persons over 65 who are entitled to benefits under the railroad retirement program and the Old-Age Survivors Disability and Health Insurance Program (OASDHI), which is better known as the social security legislation passed in 1935. The railroad retirement program was a separate program in the 1935 Social Security Act covering specific segments of the working public.[3]

Part A of Medicare covers inpatient hospital care and care in skilled nursing facilities and home health agencies following hospitalization. Part B, the supplementary medical insurance program, is the voluntary portion of Medicare in which any person eligible for Part A may enroll for a monthly premium. The monthly premium is matched by federal funds. The services covered include physician services, home health care, medical and other health services, outpatient hospital services, and various other services.[4] About 96 percent of those eligible have enrolled in Part B.[5]

HISTORY

Almost from the beginning of the 20th century the issue of government health insurance has been a heated and ongoing struggle that has pitted classic political adversaries in direct conflict. Whichever side of the fence a member of Congress happened to be on with regard to national health insurance, that member would have powerful backing. The opposition to government health insurance of any kind consisted of a mixture of Republicans and conservative southern Democrats backed by the American Medical Association (AMA) and American Hospital Association (AHA) among others, while the proponents of government health insurance were moderate and liberal Democrats backed by the AFL-CIO, along with myriad other groups representing labor and the aged.[6]

Early attempts to create some kind of national health care plan produced extremely broad proposals that had little success. Interest began to grow during the Great Depression when President Roosevelt's committee that was formulating the Social Security Act of 1935 put one line in the bill to the effect that the Social Security Agency should study the problem. This line was struck out of the final bill.[7]

Attempts after World War II to pass some type of government health insurance were countered by the AMA, which raised the spectre of "socialized medicine" and predicted doom for American medicine. In response, there was a shift in the thrust of government health proposals. They now began to focus on the aged, since this group had an obvious and easily proven problem with health care and commanded the public's sympathy. As the social security system was proposed as the method of financing most government health insurance proposals, support for the proposal began to build. One reason for this was that Social Security did not carry the stigma of a government giveaway like welfare.[8]

The Forand Bill, written by Aime J. Forand in 1957, contained all the major features of Title XVIII, which was finally passed in 1965. The King-Anderson Bill was first proposed in 1961, rewritten in 1962, and rewritten again in 1965 when it was finally accepted as Medicare.[9]

REIMBURSEMENT

An obvious concern of all health care administrators dealing with Medicare is where their institutions will get their money from and how they will get it. With respect to Medicare, the procedure of paying providers for services performed under the program involves several different organizations. Reimbursement to providers of services under Medicare is supplied on behalf of the program by public or private organizations and agencies acting as fiscal intermediaries chosen by the providers, in accordance with federal regulations. The providers are reimbursed by these intermediaries.[10]

Basically, the intermediary will make interim payments, not less than one a month, to the provider in amounts that are agreed-upon estimates determined by a procedure specified in the contract. The majority of providers are on a periodic interim payment (PIP) program that provides for biweekly payments for estimated volumes of activity. Generally, the provider will submit to the intermediary actual costs and volumes of activity on a quarterly schedule on which interim payments are based. Hospitals in particular are reimbursed on a per diem basis for inpatients and are billed charges for outpatients. At the end of an accounting period, the actual cost of Medicare services is determined and a final settlement is made retroactively. Physicians and agencies are reimbursed on the basis of usual and customary charges for their services.[11]

In formulating methods for making fair reimbursement for services rendered to beneficiaries of Medicare, payment is made on the basis of current costs of the individual provider, rather than costs of a past period or at a fixed negotiated rate. This provides for flexibility in reimbursement to protect the provider from being disadvantaged in changing situations. All payments to providers must be based upon the "reasonable cost" of services under Title XVIII of the Social Security Act and must be related to the care of beneficiaries. Reasonable cost includes all necessary and proper costs incurred in rendering covered services.[12]

About 90 percent of contracts covering Part A of Medicare (hospital insurance) is held by Blue Cross Association as an intermediary. Since providers choose their own intermediaries, Blue Cross had the advantage of having dealt extensively with hospitals. The intermediaries for Part B (supplementary medical insurance) of Medicare are selected by the Secretary of the Department of Health and Human Services (HHS). Blue Shield plans hold about 60 percent of these contracts, with the other 40 percent going to commercial insurance companies.[13]

The uniformity of the administration of the Medicare program is in direct contrast to the Medicaid program, where reimbursement procedures are worked out by each state. Each state determines "reasonable cost." Payments for medical care and services are made directly to medical practitioners and other suppliers, or they can be made through a fiscal intermediary. Each state may choose its own method, as long as it meets federal specifications.[14]

THE TRACK RECORD

Let us now examine the track record of Medicare to see just what it has accomplished and where it has failed. Medicare went into effect in July, 1966, and right from the start benefit payments outstripped actuarial projections. During its first year, the program cost $400 million more than predicted. In 1975, outlays exceeded original projections by 100 percent.[15]

Despite these cost overruns, Medicare seems to have been generally successful in accomplishing its goal of extending to all the aged in this country insurance coverage that before was available only to the small percentage who could afford it. Surveys done under contract to the Social Security Administration during Medicare's first two years of operation indicated increased utilization and increased availability of health care to the aged. The immediate impact of the Medicare program on the utilization of covered services seemed to four-fold: (1) short-term hospital use rose 25 percent, measured by days of care per enrolled aged person; (2) inpatient medical services increased commensurately; (3) use of long-term medical institutions did not change, but it shifted to institutions covered by Medicare; (4) the proportion of persons using ambulatory medical services remained about the same. [16]

Medicare has also facilitated some improvement of institutional conditions due to accreditation requirements, encouraged development of cost analysis and control programs, and made professional review (e.g., PSROs) a requirement.[17]

Medicare of course has many shortcomings. It does not cover many services that can be very expensive, such as out-of-hospital prescription drugs or hearing aids. Deductibles, coinsurance, and Part-B premiums are steadily rising, and in many states these must be paid for by the beneficiaries. Patients must also pay physician fees, which are not deemed "reasonable" by the Medicare intermediary. Today, Medicare covers only about 80 percent of an aged person's total bill.[18]

From the provider point of view, Medicare is a mixed blessing. While providing for cost reimbursement for what would otherwise be charity cases, the Medicare load on providers has resulted in a heavy "loss" of funds available for replacement of assets, since inflation renders reimbursement relatively inadequate on an historical cost basis. Given rising governmental expenditures through the Medicare program, the providers are faced with cost containment through reimbursement mechanisms that put limits on utilization and on routine costs per day. The hospital is not reimbursed for increasing costs that are deemed unnecessary for the care of the patient, such as telephone expenses, physician office space, and revenues from parking lots.

Such concerns, compounded by similarities in the Medicaid program, have caused health care administrators to seek alternatives to the reimbursement mechanisms presently in place. One such alternative is state-administered prospective rate review systems.

MEDICARE PROCEDURES

The Medicare program provides for periodic, per diem reimbursement to hospitals through the year for inpatients and for 80 percent of charges for outpatients and hospital-based physician services (both reimbursements are net of patient deductibles). Medicare also provides for biweekly payments to hospitals via the periodic interim payment program (PIP). The mechanics of PIP are as follows:

- Quarterly, the hospital submits to Medicare its total costs of operations on a cumulative basis and on gross patient-day experience.

- The hospital also submits cumulative numbers of Medicare patient days for the corresponding time frame.

- Medicare then divides the expenses by the number of total patient days to arrive at a per diem.

- Adjustments are made to this per diem for the historic percentage of outpatient costs, average deductibles, and cost adjustments for other revenue and nonallowable costs.
- This computed net per diem is then multiplied by the annualized number of Medicare patient days and then divided by 26 (the number of biweekly periods in a year) to arrive at the PIP payment to the hospital.
- If the payment increases, the hospital receives a lump-sum settlement. If the payment decreases, the hospital pays Medicare for the historic overpayment.
- When the hospital is to receive payment for a particular Medicare patient, no check is received for inpatients. Rather, payment is made via a voucher listing the patient's information and gross charges, nonallowable services, deductible and coinsurance, and per diem amount paid. The difference between the per diem plus deductibles and coinsurance amounts and the gross charges is the contractual allowance.

Figure 4–1 indicates the data flow in Medicare reimbursement procedures. Note the relationship of the Medicare log and cost reporting functions as a reporting cycle somewhat separate from the regular accounting cycle. The tie between the cost reporting functions and regular accounting operations is generally made through adjusting journal entries at the time of the preparation of the Medicare cost report.

To illustrate the internal relationship of the prepayment process to the hospital accounting system, consider the following accounting data and journal entries.

The chart of accounts entries applicable to the Medicare prepayment process are indicated below.

Account Number	Description	Classification
100–00	Regular cash	Asset
110–00	Accounts receivable	Asset
220–00	PIP clearing	Liability
570–00	Medicare allowance	Revenue deduction
550–00+	Various revenue accounts	Revenue

Following are the journal entries to record Medicare prepayment transactions.

The hospital receives a $200,000 biweekly PIP check. The following entries are made:

Entry Code	Date	Account No.	Description	Debit	Credit
CR–1	5/2/79	100–00	Regular cash	$200,000	
		220–00	PIP clear		$200,000

Figure 4-1 Medicare System Data Flow

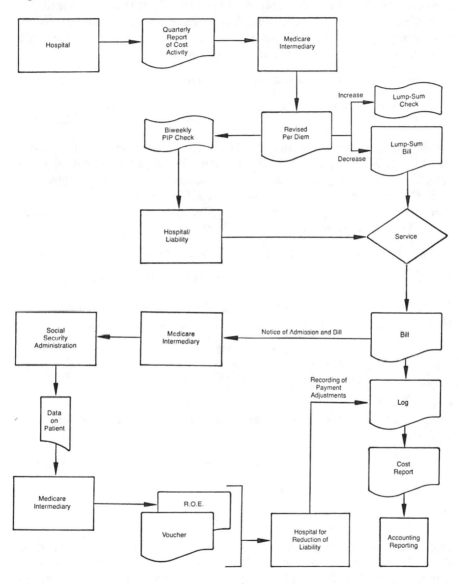

Note the establishment here of the liability created by the receipt of the PIP advance. Payment has been made with the service yet to be performed.

A Medicare patient, Gerda Jean, has incurred charges totalling $10,000 during a 15-day stay at the hospital. To record the revenue associated with services provided, the following entries are recorded:

Entry Code	Date	Account No.	Description	Debit	Credit
Rev-1	5/5/79	110-00	Accts. rec.	$10,000	
		550-00	Revenue		$10,000

Note the establishment of the receivable and associated revenue. At this point in the Medicare cycle, the billing would be prepared and entries made into the Medicare log. This step will be discussed later in this chapter.

The current per diem for the hospital is $200 per Medicare day (this per diem varies from hospital to hospital.) The deductible for this patient is $160. The following voucher is received by the hospital:

Patient Name	Days	Gross Charges	Per Diem × Days	Deductible	Paid
Gerda Jean	15	$10,000	$200 × 15 = $3,000	$160	$2,840

The data on this transaction may be analyzed as follows (remember that under the PIP program, only a voucher is received—no check).

Gross charges	$10,000
Medicare payment	(2,840)
Patient portion	(160)
Medicare allowance	$7,000 Contractual Allowance

The following entries may now be made to record the receipt of the voucher from Medicare:

Entry Code	Date	Account No.	Description	Debit	Credit
CR-2	6/25/79	220-00	PIP clearing	$2,840	
		570-00	Medicare allowance	$7,000	
		110-00	Accts. rec.		$9,840

Note that the liability account for the PIP biweekly payment has been reduced by the amount of the voucher "payment," an allowance has been established for the difference between the gross charges and the Medicare "payment" plus the patient's deductible, and the receivable from the patient has been reduced to the $160 balance due ($10,000 − $9,840).

As a result of the second quarter PIP update, the hospital receives a check for $100,000 for prior applications of claims. In analyzing this transaction, note that allowances have been overstated due to the increase in allowable

Medicare costs. Therefore, the following entry is appropriate to record receipt of the second quarter Medicare lump-sum settlement:

Entry Code	Date	Account No.	Description	Debit	Credit
CR–3	7/3/79	100–00	Regular cash	$100,000	
		570–00	Medicare allow.		$100,000

If a payment has been due to Medicare, cash would have been credited and Medicare allowances debited for the understatement in the prior recording of Medicare allowances.

Hospital-Based Physicians

The increased size and complexity of hospitals have resulted in the addition of physicians for the operation of key ancillary services of the hospital. The physician's obligations to the institution generally include some administrative duties in departmental operations in addition to primary responsibilities in the provision of patient services. For example, the departmental radiologist may attend departmental meetings, evaluate purchases, and provide departmental inservice education. These functions would be a part of the radiologist's compensation, in addition to that from the performance of patient-related duties. Via the 1967 amendments to the Social Security Act, Medicare provided for the combined billing option for the hospital inpatient services of radiologists and pathologists and for all hospital outpatient departments except psychiatric services, effective April 1, 1968. The combined billing option allows the hospital to bill Medicare for hospital-based physicians on a direct basis as a percentage of billed charges or as an amount per test. Administrative services to the hospital performed by the physician are reimbursable under Part A of Medicare and are therefore reimbursable as full inpatient costs. The remainder of the physician's compensation is outpatient-related and reimbursable on an 80 percent basis as Part B costs.

In electing the combined billing option, all physicians within a particular department must agree to combined billing procedures, allowing the hospital to bill and collect; and the compensation arrangements between the provider and the provider-based physician must be either fixed compensation (e.g., salary) or a percentage of charges. Fee-for-service arrangements are specifically excluded from the combined billing and cost report settlement option (this exclusion results in a separate physician billing and the payment of reasonable and customary charges without cost report options). Hospitals must maintain and submit to the Medicare intermediary physician rationales (Medicare Form GC 744). The purpose of this is to notify Medicare of the physician compensation arrangement, the percentages of Part-A and Part-B time, and the amount of estimated compensation and gross charges. The procedure is illustrated in the following example.

The departmental radiologist is paid 30 percent of gross charges. Generally, 40 percent of the radiologist's time is spent on administrative duties and 60 percent is spent on patient-related activities. A Part-B optional billing percentage would then be calculated as $.30 \times .60 = .18$ of gross charges. Thus 18 percent of gross departmental charges must be billed as Part B on the Medicare billing for each patient billed under the combined billing. Therefore, the inpatient Medicare bill would reflect 82 percent of gross charges as radiology and 18 percent as the Part-B physician component. For cost reporting purposes, 40 percent of the radiologist's compensation would be Part A (inpatient) and 60 percent Part B.

Regardless of the percentage of Part-A and Part-B services, radiology and pathology are reimbursed under Part A of Medicare and, as such, full allowable costs are reimbursed. However, the Part-B components of other hospital-based physicians are reimbursed at 80 percent of allowable costs.

From the above discussion it can be readily seen that it is extremely important for the hospital to spell out the specific method of physician contract reimbursement, citing, for example, salary, percentage of charges, or fee for service, as well as the duties and administrative responsibilities, in order to support the Part-A and Part-B percentage determinations.

Billing and Log Procedures

When inpatient services are provided to a Medicare patient, it is necessary to file with Medicare for a report of eligibility (ROE). A notice of admission is sent to the Medicare intermediary who forwards the notice to the Social Security Administration. The data received from Medicare via the ROE are necessary for billing purposes.

Once the ROE is received by the hospital, a bill for services may be prepared. Inpatient billings for Part-A services are made via Form SSA 1453 (6). While services are being provided to a Medicare patient, the hospital is required to maintain an active utilization review committee to review the patient's stay and to compare treatments and lengths of stay with standards for the diagnosis. The attending physician is required to certify for the stay and to recertify periodically during the stay. If stays are beyond approved limits or if noncovered services are performed, the hospital must notify the patient in writing of the fact that Medicare will not pay for the service and that the patient is liable for payment. If this notice is not given, the patient may not be billed for the noncovered service.

Part-B physician components of a hospital service are billed on Form SSA 1554 (2); the physician rationales determine the appropriate portions of the hospital bill for physician's service that are billed on this form. Outpatient services are billed on Form SSA 1483. The key elements of the billing forms relate to a breakdown of services by routine, special care, and ancillary areas. It is essential that the hospital analyze the details of this aspect to determine that the specific charges flowing to the billing areas best represent classifications on a uniform basis consistent with cost data.

The hospital must also ensure that the information on the billing forms is complete and accurate. Simple errors can result in substantial delays in information flow. It is also essential that the Medicare patients or their agents authorize billings to Medicare. The signature of the patient or agent is required on all billing forms.

The data on the billing form must be summarized in a detailed listing of Medicare activity on what is known as the Medicare log. There are many ways to maintain this log, but the general practice is to identify Medicare patients upon admission or registration in outpatient and emergency room areas and to record the date of initial contact and the number and name of the patient in the log. In billing, a copy of the billing forms is sent to the log area, where detailed routine and ancillary services and related gross covered charges are entered for each patient. Upon receipt of the voucher or payment from Medicare, the detailed information corresponding to the entry for the initial billing is recorded in the log. At this time, appropriate adjustments may be made to the log to correct any errors discovered in the payment process.

Medicare Data Flow and Cost Reporting

The hospital maintains throughout the year the log of Medicare patients and the departmentalized, ancillary services provided to Medicare patients on a gross charge basis. At the end of the fiscal year, the hospital prepares a cost report that shows the allocation of allowable costs to revenue producing cost centers, for example, routine care, intensive care unit (ICU), laboratory, radiology. Once the allocation of all costs has been completed, a cost-to-charge ratio is computed for each ancillary area. For example:

Radiology:	Full cost	$1,000,000	
	Charges to all patients	$2,000,000	
	Cost-to-charge ratio	$\dfrac{\$1,000,000}{\$2,000,000}$	= 0.5

The cost-to-charge ratio is then applied to Medicare charges, and the cost for provision of each ancillary service to Medicare patients is computed:

Radiology:			
		Medicare charges	$500,000
	×	Cost-to-charge ratio	× 0.5
		Radiology Medicare cost	$250,000

This procedure applies to both inpatient and outpatient ancillary services.

Inpatient routine and special-care units are reimbursed on a per-day basis. The procedure includes the following ten steps:

1. From the full-cost allocation, the cost of routine services is identified.
2. Salaries for the provision of general care are next identified. These are the direct nursing salaries associated with routine care.
3. Total patient days are accumulated for all patients in routine, general care (not special units such as ICU).
4. Patient days for aged (over 65), pediatric, and maternity patients are accumulated.
5. Total costs minus salary costs are then divided by the total patient days of all patients.
6. Direct routine salary costs are divided by total patient days of all patients.
7. The per diem salary costs computed in Step 6 are multiplied by the sum of aged, pediatric, and maternity days. This total is then multiplied by 8.5 percent to determine the 8.5 percent differential applicable to more intense nursing care for these categories of patients.
8. The salary costs plus the differential are added together and divided by total patient days to arrive at an allowable per day salary cost.
9. The per diems arrived at in Steps 5 and 8 are added together to compute the Medicare routine cost per diem (which must be below the allowable routine cost limitation).
10. Medicare days from the log are then multiplied by the per diem of Step 9 to compute allowable Medicare costs from routine services.

For special care units like ICUs, per diem costs are computed by dividing the total special-care patient days of all patients into the full cost of the unit. No adjustment is made for nursing differentials. The computed per diem costs are then multiplied by the number of special-care Medicare days for the computation of allowable Medicare costs from special-care services.

Medicare costs from all inpatient areas are accumulated from the above computations and are compared with the billed charges for Medicare services. At the present time, Medicare pays the lower of costs or charges.

Allowable reimbursable expenses are then compared to interim payments made to the hospital. Any excess cost is paid by Medicare and becomes a receivable; likewise, any excess amounts from interim payments are payable to Medicare. At this point, the reader should refer again to the flow of data in the hospital's Medicare system shown in Figure 4–1.

The interfacing of the Medicare system and the hospital's accounting system is made via adjusting journal entries after the cost report has been prepared. The following entries illustrate the relationship of accounting procedures and Medicare cost reporting and settlements.

The following chart of accounts entries are recorded:

Account Number	Description	Classification
100–00	Regular cash	Asset
220–00	PIP clearing	Liability
570–00	Medicare allowance	Revenue deduction
120–00	Medicare receivable	Asset
220–01	Medicare payable	Liability
110–01	Reserve for Medicare allow.	Contra-Asset

To determine the appropriate journal entries, suppose that the allowable Medicare costs computed via the Medicare cost report are $2,500,000 and biweekly PIP payments total $2,000,000. The receivable from Medicare is then $500,000 ($2,500,000 − $2,000,000). An analysis of this transaction results in the conclusion that interim per diems were understated by $500,000 and that Medicare allowances were overstated by $500,000. Therefore, to record the receivable computed by the 1979 Medicare cost report, the adjusting journal entry is:

Entry Code	Date	Account No.	Description	Debit	Credit
AJE–1	1/3/80	120–00	Medicare receivable	$500,000	
		570–00	Medicare allowance		$500,000

Note that, if interim payments had exceeded costs, a liability would have been established.

The cost report must be prepared on an accrual basis. Therefore, all outstanding Medicare days must be reflected in the hospital's accounts, particularly at the end of the fiscal year. Suppose that the hospital had 1,000 Medicare days outstanding, gross covered charges of $300,000, a current per diem of $200 per day, and deductibles and coinsurance of $50,000. Suppose further that the 220–00 account (PIP clearing) has a balance of $125,000.

(Payment for days will be made at the per diem in effect at the time of service.) An analysis of these data shows the following:

Gross charges	$300,000
Days × per diem	
1,000 × $200	(200,000)
Deductibles and coinsurance	(50,000)
Computed allowance	$50,000
Days × pier diem	$200,000
Deductibles and coinsurance	(50,000)
Computed PIP bal.	$150,000
PIP bal. per bks.	(125,000)
Required adjustment	$25,000

To record the computed allowance for outstanding Medicare days at 12/31/79, the following entries are made:

Entry Code	Date	Account No.	Description	Debit	Credit
AJE–2	1/3/80	570–00	Medicare allowance	$50,000	
		110–00	Reserve for Medicare		$50,000

The usual procedure is to record allowances at the time of payment or receipt of a voucher. As a result, the receivables balance in the accounts must reflect a reserve or reduction from gross receivables for the estimated uncollectable balance, in the above instance, the 110–00 reserve for Medicare allowances, which has a credit balance and is classified as a contra-asset account reflecting a reduction of the asset balance in accounts receivables. To bring the PIP clearing account balance to the computed balance for Medicare days outstanding at 12/31/79, the following is recorded:

Entry Code	Date	Account No.	Description	Debit	Credit
AJE–3	1/3/80	570–00	Medicare allowance	$25,000	
		220–00	PIP clearing		$25,000

At this point, the accounts reflect the complete Medicare accounting cycle. It is important that the balance of the Medicare-related accounts be reconciled periodically throughout the year to ensure a continuance of accuracy in the computations and recordings. External confirmation of Medicare activity is available via log, voucher, and account reconciliations and comparisons to summary reports supplied by Medicare.

The basic issues in the preparation of a cost report are the identification of full costs for services rendered to Medicare patients and the determination of the costs applicable to Medicare, based on the percentage of Medicare charges to total charges on a department-by-department basis. To identify the full costs of operating a department, one must allocate all overhead costs to the revenue producing departments. Medicare recognizes the single-cost step-down—among more sophisticated methodologies—for this process. Under this approach, overhead items such as depreciation, operation of plant, administration, and dietary are allocated to other areas based on appropriate statistics. The following simplified example presents a concise picture of the cost reporting process.

Statistics

	Sq. Ft.	Salaries	Pr. Days
Employee health and welfare	1,000	$15,000	
Dietary	5,000	50,000	
Administration and general	1,000	45,000	
X-ray	4,000	15,000	
Laboratory	5,000	10,000	
General care	25,000	40,000	15,000

	Total Revenue	Medicare Revenue	Medicare Days
X-ray	$ 150,000	$100,000	
Lab.	250,000	100,000	
General care	1,500,000	600,000	6,000
Total Days: 15,000			

Given the above data, the reader should now

• Determine the full cost of x-ray, laboratory, and general care, using the single cost step-down procedure.

• Determine the Medicare reimbursement for each area and in total.

• Determine the contractual allowance.

From the data provided below, the reader should now calculate the effect a 20 percent increase in rates would have.

	Direct Costs	Allocation Base
Depreciation	$1,000,000	Sq. Ft.
Employee health and welfare	100,000	Salaries
Dietary	500,000	Pt. Days

Administration and general	50,000	Accum. Cost
X-ray	20,000	—
Laboratory	15,000	—
General care	100,000	—
	$1,785,000	

The allocation of depreciation costs is based on the number of square feet contained in the departments listed below depreciation on the step-down chart. To determine how much should be allocated to each of the departments, the following method is used.

$$\frac{\text{Direct Cost of Depreciation}}{\text{Sum of Department's sq. ft.}} =$$

$$\frac{1,000,000}{41,000} = \$24.390244 \text{ per sq. ft.}$$

This ratio is then multiplied by each department's square footage to obtain how much of the cost of depreciation should be allocated to each of the remaining departments.

Employee Health and Welfare	1,000 × 24.390244	=	$24,390.24
Dietary	5,000 × "	=	121,951.22
Admin. & Gen.	1,000 × "	=	24,390.24
X-ray	4,000 × "	=	97,560.98
Lab.	5,000 × "	=	121,951.22
General Care	25,000 × "	=	609,756.10

The allocation of the costs of the Employee Health and Welfare department must be made among the remaining departments on the step-down. This is done on the basis of the salaries of the departments below Employee Health and Welfare on the step-down. First, the sum of the salaries for all the departments is figured. This equals $175,000. The salaries for Employee Health and Welfare, which total $15,000, are subtracted from this, leaving $160,000 for the denominator. The numerator comes from the costs of Employee Health and Welfare which totals $124,390.24 (direct cost plus the previous allocation of depreciation). This equals $0.777439. This means that for every $1.00 of salary a department has, it receives $0.777439 of Employee Health and Welfare. The breakdown is as follows:

Dietary	$50,000 × 0.777439	=	$38,871.950
Admin. & Gen.	$45,000 × "	=	$34,984.755
X-ray	$15,000 × "	=	$11,661.585
Lab.	$10,000 × "	=	$ 7,774.390
General Care	$40,000 × "	=	$31,097.560

The allocation of the costs of the dietary department is based on the number of patient days of each department. There is only one department that has any patient days, so all Dietary costs are allocated to General Care.

The allocation of the costs of Administration and General are figured on the basis of the accumulated costs of the remaining departments, using the costs of Administration and General as the numerator and the sum of the costs of the departments below it on the step-down as the denominator. This yields 0.0652742. This ratio is multiplied by the accumulated costs for each of the remaining departments, then is allocated to it. The breakdown is as follows:

X-ray	$ 129,222.57 × 0.0652742	= $ 8,434.8936
Lab.	$ 144,725.61 × "	= $ 9,446.8414
General Care	$1,401,676.80 × "	= $91,493.2640

The answer to part 1 of the problem is:

The full costs of X-ray, Laboratory, and General Care by using the single-cost step-down are:

X-ray	$ 137,657.46
Lab.	$ 154,172.45
General Care	$1,493,170.10

To find the Medicare reimbursement of each area and the total, take the total cost of each ancillary and divide it by the total charges for that department.

$$\text{X-ray:} \quad \frac{137,657.46}{150,000} = 0.9171164$$

$$\text{Laboratory:} \quad \frac{154,172.45}{250,000} = 0.6166898$$

Then multiply the resulting ratios by Medicare revenue associated with each department

X-ray:	0.9171164 × 100,000 = $91,771.64
Lab.:	0.6166898 × 100,000 = $61,668.98

Total ancillary Medicare costs = $153,440.62

The routine costs or general care costs for Medicare reimbursement will now be figured. Take the cost associated with General Care from the step-down and divide it by the total number of patient days.

$$\$1,493,170.10 \div 15,000 = \$99.544673 \text{ per day}$$

Then multiply this per diem by the number of Medicare days.

$$\$99.544673 \times 6,000 = \$597,268.04$$

Then add this figure to the costs associated with the ancillary departments.

X-ray	$ 91,771.64
Laboratory	$ 61,668.98
Total Ancillary	$153,440.62
General Care	$597,268.04
Total M/C Costs	$750,708.66

The Medicare per diem is $750,708.66 ÷ 6000 = $125.1181.
To determine the contractual allowance, total the Medicare charges:

X-ray	$100,000
Lab.	100,000
General Care	600,000
Total	$800,000

Take the total charge and subtract from it the total Medicare costs.

$$\$800,000 - \$750,708.66 = \$49,291.34$$

This figure, $49,291.34, is the contractual allowance.

If there is a 20 percent increase in the rates this will change the Medicare reimbursement and the contractual allowance in the following way.

Total Revenue

X-ray	$ 150,000 × 1.2 = $ 180,000
Lab.	$ 250,000 × 1.2 = $ 300,000
General Care	$1,500,000 × 1.2 = $1,800,000
Total	$1,900,000 × 1.2 = $2,280,000

Medicare Revenue

X-ray	$100,000 × 1.2 = $120,000
Lab.	$100,000 × 1.2 = $120,000
General Care	$600,000 × 1.2 = $720,000
Total	$800,000 × 1.2 = $960,000

The ratios for the ancillaries are:

$$\text{X-ray:} \quad \frac{137,657.46}{180,000} = 0.7647637$$

Lab.: $\dfrac{154,172.45}{300,000}$ = 0.5139082

The ratios are then applied to the revenues for the Medicare patients.

X-ray: 0.7647637 × 120,000 = $91,771.64
Lab.:   0.5139082 × 120,000 = 61,668.98

The Medicare reimbursement for the ancillaries remains as it was before the increase in revenue because there was no corresponding increase in costs incurred by the hospital.

However, the contractual allowance will be different because the total Medicare revenue has increased to $960,000. From this figure is subtracted the same figure for total costs, which is $750,708.66. This yields a figure of $209,291.34. This allowance will have to be returned to Medicare if Medicare has already paid the total revenue amount based on the past. In effecting cash flow it would supply a more favorable one during the year as Medicare pays in installments, but at the end of the period when the adjustment is made that hospital would have to come up with more money than if there were no increase in revenue.

NOTES

1. *A Discursive Dictionary of Health Care* (Washington D.C.: U.S. Government Printing Office, 1976), p. 102.

2. *Medicaid, Medicare: Which is Which?* (U.S. Department of Health, Education, and Welfare, 1971).

3. *A Discursive Dictionary of Health Care* (Washington D.C.: U.S. Government Printing Office, 1976), p. 112.

4. Ibid., p. 158.

5. Karen Davis, *National Health Insurance: Benefits, Costs and Consequences* (New York: Brookings Institution, 1975), p. 48.

6. Theodore Marmor, *The Politics of Medicare* (Chicago: Aldine Publishing Co., 1973), p. 24.

7. Ibid., p. 7–9.

8. Ibid., p. 16–20.

9. Eugene Feingold, *Medicare: Policy and Politics* (San Francisco: Chandler Publishing Co., 1966), p. 101.

10. *Principles of Reimbursement for Provider Costs and for Services By Hospital-Based Physicians* (U.S. Department of Health, Education, and Welfare, 1971), Para. 405.401.

11. Ibid., Para. 405.405.

12. Ibid., Para. 405.451.

13. Bruce L. R. Smith and Niel Hollander, *The Administration of Medicare: A Shared Responsibility* (Washington, D.C.: National Academy of Public Administration Foundation, 1973), pp. 3–5.

14. *Medicare and Medicaid Guide: 1973 S.S. and Medicare Explained* (Chicago: Commerce Clearing House, 1972), p. 399.

15. Larry Frederick, *"Ten Years of Medicare and Medicaid," Medical World News* 16 (March 10, 1975): 60.

16. Arthur E. Hess, "A Ten Year Perspective on Medicare," *Public Health Reports* 91: 299–302.

17. Ibid., p. 300.

18. Frederick, "Ten Years", p. 64.

19. Ibid., p. 62.

20. Lowenstein, "Early Effects of Medicare on the Health Care of the Aged," *Social Security Bulletin,* April 1971, p. 3.

21. Avedis Donabedian, "Effects of Medicare and Medicaid on the Access to and the Quality of Health Care," *Public Health Reports,* July 1976, p. 30.

22. Hauge and Appel, "Utilization Data for Senior Citizens," *Hospitals,* December 1976, pp. 48–49.

23. Ibid.

24. Gornick, "Ten Years of Medicare: Impact on the Covered Population," Social Security Bulletin, July 1976, p. 8.

25. Lowenstein, "Early Effects," pp. 3–4.

26. Ibid., p. 3.

27. Donabedian, "Effects," p. 326.

28. Ibid., p. 327.

29. Ibid.

30. Ibid.

31. Hess, "A Ten Year Perspective," p. 302.

Chapter 5

The Statement of Revenues and Expenses

INTRODUCTION

The statement of revenues and expenses provides a summary review of the results of operations for a particular reporting period. In the present chapter, we will reexamine the statement of revenues and expenses of Community Medical Center for the two years ending December 31, 1977, and December 31, 1978. This statement is reproduced as Exhibit 5–1, with five major sections identified by number for discussion purposes. In this reexamination, the systems issues presented in Chapter 3 will serve as particularly useful reference points.

The five major sections are—(1) gross revenue, (2) revenue deductions, (3) other operating revenue, (4) operating expenses, and (5) nonoperating revenue and expense. Our discussion of these components will be followed by an analysis of key managerial issues related to the statement of revenues and expenses of Community Medical Center.

Figure 5–1 depicts the relationship of the financial cycles discussed in Chapter 3 to the preparation of the statement of revenues and expenses. The hospital administrator must become familiar with the illustrated data flow into the statement in order to form impressions of the results of the institution's operations. It is also important that the administration of the hospital set basic guidelines for reporting variances in these key areas.

THEORETICAL DEFINITIONS

Revenues are generally created as a result of selling goods and/or services to others. In the final analysis of business operations, assets are placed into

Exhibit 5-1 Community Medical Center: Statements of Revenues and Expenses, for the Years 1977 and 1978 Ending December 31

Section		1978	1977
		(in 000s)	
1.	Operating Revenue:		
	Gross revenue from patient services:		
	Inpatient	$14,513	$12,468
	Outpatient	1,458	1,303
		$15,971	$13,771
2.	Revenue deductions	1,510	1,599
	Net revenue from patient services	$14,461	$12,172
3.	Other operating revenue	222	179
	Total operating revenue	$14,683	$12,351
4.	Operating Expenses:		
	Salaries	$ 7,045	$ 5,773
	Fees and commissions	1,379	1,193
	Supplies	2,748	2,103
	Other expenses	1,753	1,178
	Interest and amortization of debt expense	520	549
	Depreciation-cost	1,125	1,139
	Total operating expenses	$14,570	$11,935
	Income (loss) from operations	$ 113	$ 416
5.	Nonoperating Revenue:		
	Contributions	21	9
	Interest income	143	149
	Excess (deficiency) of revenues over expenses	$ 277	$ 574

Figure 5-1 Financial Cycle Interface with the Statement of Revenues and Expenses

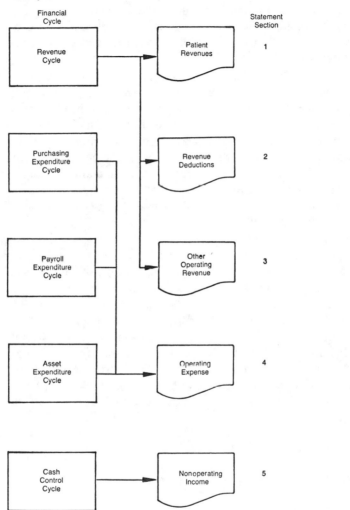

the operations of the enterprise with the expectation of increasing the volume and/or value of these assets or, possibly, of reducing the liabilities of the concern. Simply put, an increase in assets or a decrease in liabilities results in an increase in the equity or fund balance of the institution. The increase in the fund balance is known as an excess of revenues over expenses. Basically, expenses are assets that are consumed in the operations of an institution to provide goods or services resulting in revenue. The transfer of assets to expenses and the increase in the fund balance of excess revenue results in revenues having credit balances and expenses having debit balances. The basic accounting equation is assets = liabilities + fund balance, where an increase in assets must be offset by an increase in liabilities or the fund balance.

One of the fundamental accounting principles governing the preparation of the statement of revenues and expenses on an accrual basis is that revenues generated for a given period must be matched to the expenses consumed in the generation of these revenues in the same time period. Generally, the financial statements of a hospital are prepared on an accrual basis. The implication of this matching principle is the need to recognize revenue at the time of the provision of the service, to make allowances for potential uncollectable accounts, to recognize capital asset usage via depreciation and depletion, and to allocate all expenses to the period associated with their consumption in the generation of revenue.

The accrual basis provides for a better recognition of the results of operations of the institution, compared with the cash basis of accounting, which recognizes revenues and expenses at the time of collection or payment. Thus, the present discussion will focus on accrual accounting.

Accounting practices must be applied on a uniform and consistent basis. Without accounting and reporting consistency between accounting periods, comparisons and managerial information would be distorted. An example of this distortion would be the case of a change from a straight line method of depreciation to an accelerated method. Such a change in practice would result in either an increase or a decrease in expense, depending on the life position of the institution's overall capital assets.

MAJOR SECTIONS

Section 1: Gross Patient Revenue

At the time of provision of service to a patient, a receivable is created and a charge is made for the service. The charge for each service must be reported by area of service to a central location for incorporation in the billing and collection system. The general journal entry format is:

	Debit	Credit
Accounts receivable	xxxx.xx	
Revenue		xxxx.xx

Note the increase of an asset and the recording of the related increase as revenue. To enhance managerial decision making, revenue should be reported on a gross basis, separate from bad debts and other revenue deductions. A netting of revenues and deductions would result in the loss of important information on patient service activity and of the full effect of deductions on the revenue-generation capacity of the institution.

It is the responsibility of the hospital's administration to set policies regarding items and services to be charged for and the rates to be charged. Charges should be set at a level to provide an adequate return for replacement of assets and for necessary expansions of technology in line with projected costs and activity levels. Actual revenues by service area should be compared with planned or budgeted levels and variances investigated. Actions should be taken where appropriate to ensure adherence to managerial policies.

Comparisons to prior year levels provide valuable information regarding trends in hospital activity by service. However, care must be taken to ensure that increases in rates between periods are discounted. If they are not, increases in revenue may lead to a conclusion that activity has increased while in fact activity levels may have actually declined, with the rate increases accounting for the increase in revenue. Strict dollar comparisons of revenue provide only a partial picture of the activity of the institution. It is imperative that statistics of activity by service area be incorporated into the managerial component of the revenue cycle and be related to revenues generated to ensure full collection of revenue for service and to facilitate identification of possible trends toward more complex and higher charge services.

Section 2: Revenue Deductions

One of the unique operating practices of a hospital is the provision of service to patients regardless of private ability to pay or of coverage by third party payers. The related diversity of payment methods results in several possible types of revenue deductions. In the case of contractual allowances related to Medicare, the difference between Medicare gross charges and the cost of Medicare services plus the patient's portion of the bill—deductibles and coinsurance—is the amount of the allowance. Blue Cross inpatient reimbursement allows for a cost-plus 5 percent payment to the hospital. The difference between gross charges and reimbursement is a revenue deduction that is the contractual allowance. Many state Medicaid program payments are also on a cost basis, again resulting in a contractual allowance. Basic accounting entries related to contractual allowances are indicated below:

	Debit	Credit
Revenue deduction	xxxx.xx	
Accts. rec.		xxxx.xx

Note the reduction of the asset and the corresponding debit to the revenue deduction area.

The reduction in accounts receivables for allowances for unpaid accounts is made via a contra-asset account as a reserve for allowances. The entry in this case is:

	Debit	Credit
Revenue deduction	xxxx.xx	
Reserve for allow.		xxxx.xx

Again, note the reduction of the asset and the debit to the allowance as the revenue deduction.

The preparation of a cost report on an interim basis is a difficult and time-consuming task. However, most allowances are recorded at the time of payment, leaving an amount of uncollectable funds in the accounts receivable area throughout the year until the cost report is prepared. Therefore, the amount of estimated allowances must be computed on an interim basis. A simple formula to use in the estimation of the allowance is (gross charges + other operating revenue + nonoperating revenue − expenses) × percentage of cost reimbursement activity = estimated contractual allowances. The result is then compared to the amount on the "books," and the following entry is made for the difference:

		Debit	Credit
If the amount computed is under book levels:	Reserve for Allowances	xxxx.xx	
	Revenue Deduction		xxxx.xx
If the amount computed is over book levels:	Revenue Deduction	xxxx.xx	
	Reserve for Allowances		xxxx.xx

The reader should compare the above estimation formula with the flows discussed in Chapter 4 on Medicare cost reporting.

In addition to contractual allowances, bad debts are a type of revenue deduction. Because of the general practice of hospitals to provide service to all patients regardless of their ability to pay, and despite the vast amount of insurance coverage commonly available, a certain portion of patients treated at a hospital have no insurance and, for one reason or another, do not pay their bills for services rendered. Consequently, some of the gross revenues reported on the statement of revenues and expenses is in the form of bad debts. In order to match revenues and expenses for the operations of a particular time period, it is necessary to estimate the amount of bad debts applicable to the reporting period and to establish reserves and allowances for the estimates. It is extremely difficult, if not impossible, to be precise in determining bad debts at the time of service to a particular patient. Therefore, estimates of the expected bad debts must be made as they pertain to the revenue generated and to the accounts carried as accounts receivable.

Procedures for estimating the amount of bad debts vary, but in all cases specific issues must be addressed. Periodically (at least once a year), a detailed review should be made of accounts by carrier and age within carrier categories. This review, usually done on a sample basis, should yield percentages of each account that are estimated to be uncollectable. Computation of percentages and dollar amounts of estimated uncollectable balances can then be done by carrier and age. As an example, consider the following case: XYZ Hospital has five classifications of accounts receivable. Balances in total and within age by date of discharge are as follows:

Company	Gross Amount	0–30 Days	31–90 Days	91–180 Days	181–1 yr.	over 1 yr.
A	$ 500,000	$200,000	$100,000	$ 75,000	$ 75,000	$ 50,000
B	300,000	100,000	75,000	50,000	50,000	25,000
Medicaid	200,000	100,000	50,000	25,000	25,000	-0-
Medicare	250,000	150,000	75,000	25,000	-0-	-0-
Self-pay	400,000	100,000	100,000	100,000	50,000	50,000
Total	$1,650,000	$650,000	$400,000	$275,000	$200,000	$125,000

From a detailed sample taken from each classification, the following analysis of the categorization of bad debts can be made, based on the formula by category.

$$\frac{\text{Estimated \% $\times$ account amount}}{\text{Account balances in the sample}}$$

Company	0–30	31–90	91–180	181–1 yr.	over 1 yr.
A	5%	10%	30%	60%	100%
B	7%	14%	40%	70%	100%
Medicaid	0%	5%	15%	25%	100%
Medicare	0%	0%	0%	5%	100%
Self-pay	7%	20%	55%	80%	100%

By multiplying average percentages of bad debts by the amounts by category, the total volume of estimated bad debts may be computed:

Company	0–30	31–90	91–180	181–1 yr.	over 1 yr.
A	$10,000	$10,000	$ 22,500	$ 45,000	$ 50,000
B	7,000	10,500	20,000	35,000	25,000
Medicaid	-0-	2,500	3,750	-0-	-0-
Medicare	-0-	-0-	-0-	-0-	-0-
Self-pay	7,000	20,000	55,000	40,000	50,000
Total	$24,000	$43,000	$101,250	$120,000	$125,000

Thus, the total amount of computed bad debts is $413,250 or ($413,250 ÷ $1,650,000) 25.04 percent of accounts receivable. Suppose that the book balance of bad debts reserves at the end of the fiscal year is $500,000. An adjustment must be made to adjust the book balance to the computed level. An analysis of the transaction yields an overstatement of $86,750 ($500,000 − $413,250) in the contra-asset reserve for bad debts and an overstatement in the bad debt allowance revenue deduction. To adjust the bad-debt-related accounts to the computed balance, the journal entry is:

	Debit	Credit
Reserve for bad debts	$86,750	
Allowance for bad debts		$86,750

The accumulation of bad debt allowances is generally made monthly, based on an historic percentage of bad debt allowances to gross charges. A cross-reference to the interim estimates of allowances may be made by computing percentages of reserves to the corresponding accounts receivable balances and comparing these to historic percentages.

To determine the related flow of accounting entries, assume that the historic percentage of bad debt allowances to gross charges is four percent and that January, 1979, gross revenues total $1,200,000. The estimated allowance would then be .04 × $1,200,000 = $48,000. The related journal entry would be:

	Debit	Credit
Allowance for bad debts	$48,000	
Reserve for bad debts		$48,000

Note the increase in both the revenue deduction and the contra-asset account.

The interim estimation of bad debt allowances provides for the establishment of a reserve for bad debts in the gross accounts receivable balance. When a specific account is identified as a bad debt, it should be eliminated from the asset account, accounts receivable. Because a reserve has been established for bad debts, the actual "writing off" of an account should reduce accounts receivable and the reserve for bad debts. Thus, if a $5,000 bill is written off, the journal entry would be:

	Debit	Credit
Reserve for bad debts	$5,000	
Accounts receivable		$5,000

Suppose that, after the account is written off, a collection agency collects the $5,000 for a collection fee of 20 percent. An analysis of this transaction results in a cash collection, a collection fee expense, and the replenishment of the reserve account for an amount that was really not a bad debt. The entry to record this transaction would be:

	Debit	Credit
Cash	$4,000	
Collection fee	$1,000	
Reserve for bad debts		$5,000

It is essential that the hospital's administration and board be directly involved in the development of credit policies that govern bad debt requirements and the use of collection agencies. Also, controls must be established to ensure strict and consistent compliance with the established guidelines for receivables management. Overall testing of revenue deductions may be made by comparing reserves to accounts receivable with trends in percentages of allowances related to gross charges. Any variance from planned and/or historic relationships should be questioned and investigated. Demographic components may have changed; for example, a plant shutdown, causing variances in deductions, may result in alteration of credit policies in the light of changing environmental circumstances. If significant environmental trends and conditions are ignored, historic percentage usage for estimates may overstate or understate deductions. The increasing amounts of revenue deductions—bad debts, contractual allowances, charity and volume discounts—must be carefully monitored by hospitals to ensure that such deductions are in line with established policies and are adequately planned for in setting rates.

Section 3: Other Operating Revenue

In the performance of patient care, a hospital provides auxiliary services that generate revenue. These services include cafeteria sales to employees; parking lot services to employees, patients, and visitors; rental of office space to physicians; and the sale of x-ray, silver, and medical records (generally copies and statistical abstracts sent to insurance companies). The provision of these services by not-for-profit hospitals and the associated revenues have recently come under close scrutiny by federal agencies, in particular the IRS and Medicare. The hospital must be assured that the revenues generated are maximized but that such activities remain within the overall area of providing patient care and not expand into unrelated activities, such as selling clothing or running various shops in the vicinity of the hospital. While these are obvious examples of unrelated activities, certain less obvious areas may present a problem, for example, selling cafeteria meals to the general public or allowing persons to park in the hospital's parking lots while shopping or going to a movie. Direct administrative involvement through policies and procedures is essential to ensure compliance with the regulations governing not-for-profit institutions.

The same controls must be built into the accounting system for other operating revenues related to the revenue cycle. Centralization of data flow is essential because of the many diverse areas from which revenue may flow. Generally, the controller has responsibility for maintaining coordination of information, with the cashiering functions handled by a cashier in the business office. Cash reconciliations and classifications of receipts are essential to proper record keeping and to the assignment of revenue to various areas. One of the most critical areas related to cash control is the cafeteria. Significant amounts of cash are collected as food is served, and a supply of change must be kept on hand. Controls must be established here to ensure proper charges for items of food and that cash is reconciled and deposited intact with the hospital's central cashier for entry into the cash control cycle. When the amount of cash is sufficiently large, cash registers should be used at the point of sale, cash balances should be independently reconciled to the register tape, and cash should be transferred intact to the central cashier. No cash should be held in the cafeteria or dietary areas when a predetermined amount is not in use as change.

Journal entries to record revenue from miscellaneous operating sources are made in the following format:

	Debit	Credit
Cash (or a receivable)	xxxx.xx	
Other operating revenue		xxxx.xx

Note the increase in the asset and the corresponding increase in the revenue account.

Care must be taken to ensure proper matching of revenue with the period in which it is earned. Suppose that, on July 1, 1979, a physician pays $12,000 to the hospital for one year's rent. The recording of the receipt of the cash as revenue in 1979 would result in an overstatement of rental income in 1979 and an understatement of revenue in 1980. The original entry in this case would be:

	Debit	Credit
Cash	$12,000	
Rental income		$12,000

But then an adjusting journal entry must be made to reduce rental income to the portion pertaining only to 1979, which is one-half of $12,000 or $6,000. The offset must be made to a liability account, deferred revenue. The entry would be:

	Debit	Credit
Rental income	$6,000	
Deferred revenue		$6,000

It can be seen that this entry increases the liability account and reduces the revenue account.

As a final note, all of the above transactions must be recorded and reported in sufficient detail to allow for managerial decision making and reporting related to Medicare and IRS requirements.

Section 4: Operating Expenses

Assets that are consumed and liabilities that are increased in the provision of services related to the operation of the hospital are classified as operating expenses. To provide sufficient detail in the statement of revenues and expenses for the purposes of decision making, a general classification of expenses—salaries, fees, supplies, miscellaneous, interest, and depreciation—is maintained. Accounting cycles that interface with these expense classifications are purchasing expenditure, payroll expenditure, and asset expenditure. The journal entry for the expense accumulation is:

	Debit	Credit
Expense	xxxx.xx	
Asset (or liability)		xxxx.xx

The result is an increased expense and a reduction in assets or increased liabilities.

Consumption of assets in a particular time frame may take the form of expenditures of cash and investments, reductions of inventories, depreciation of capital assets, or amortization of prepaid expenses. The expenditure of cash for an asset to be consumed in the current reporting period, for example, for food, x-ray film, and education, results in a reduction of the asset, cash, and an increase in operating expense, as in the following journal entry:

	Debit	Credit
Expense	xxxx.xx	
Cash		xxxx.xx

Care must be taken to ensure that procedures in effect for the cash control cycle provide for control of the classification of the expense, with regard to not only the proper major classification but also to the departmental cost center responsible for the expenditure.

Goods to be used in future accounting periods are generally classified as inventories, an asset. As goods are consumed or placed into service, the asset is reduced and expenses are increased in the following journal entry:

	Debit	Credit
Expense	xxxx.xx	
Inventories		xxxx.xx

Detailed procedures for inventory accounting will be discussed in the following chapter. However, to provide a proper perspective on expense-related accounting procedures, a summary description is presented in the following paragraphs.

Withdrawals from inventories may be recorded each time a transaction is made—a perpetual system—or recorded after a physical count of the items is made—a periodic system. The most critical factor related to inventories is the procedure followed in pricing the inventory items. The pricing policy has a direct impact on the level of the reported expenses. Generally accepted accounting principles allow for several different methods of pricing inventories. Of these methods, last-in-first-out (LIFO) and first-in-first-out (FIFO) are the most common. Under LIFO pricing, it is assumed that the last items entered into inventory are the first items placed in use. Under FIFO pricing, it is assumed that the first items placed in inventory are the first items withdrawn.

Consider the following situation:

Laboratory Inventory Transactions for January, 1978

Date	Transaction	Units	Unit Price	Extension
1/1	Beginning Bal.	0	0	0
1/15	Purchase	300	$5	$1,500
1/29	Purchase	200	6	1,200
1/30	Withdrawal	300		

The inventory balance reported at 1/31/78 will differ, depending on the method chosen. Under LIFO, there are 200 units remaining in inventory (300 + 200 − 300), and the valuation of the ending inventory is made at the earliest price for the units purchased and remaining, that is, $5. Thus, the valuation of the ending inventory under LIFO is 200 × $5 = $1,000, and the expense reported is $1,500 + $1,200 − $1,000 = $1,700. The general formula used is beginning balance + purchases or additions − ending balance = expense.

Under FIFO, there are also 200 units in inventory at 1/31/79; however, now the valuation is made for the most recent price for the number of units, here $6. Therefore, the ending valuation of the inventory is $6 × 200 = $1,200; and the expense reported is $1,500 + $1,200 − $1,200 = $1,500.

A general rule related to the managerial effects of choosing between LIFO and FIFO methods is that, during periods of inflation, LIFO pricing results in higher expense and lower inventory valuation than FIFO. The reverse is true in periods of deflation. Note that in periods of inflation, LIFO, through its effect on expense, results in a higher cost for cost reimbursement and increased cash flow.

As the above discussion makes clear, it is essential that detailed records be kept of each addition to inventory on a unit price basis. If a periodic inventory pricing method is used, an adjustment must be made to inventory levels and expenses at the time of the physical inventory. Under perpetual systems, entries must be made at the time of withdrawal of the items. Control procedures to verify reported balances should be established to allow for physical inventories at least once a year.

Capital assets include all expenditures over a certain amount and with an estimated life of more than one or two years. Generally, significant item categorizations are buildings, building service equipment, fixed equipment, major movable equipment, land improvements, and land. All of these categories, with the exception of land, are depreciable assets.

To match revenues and expenses, some method must be devised to allocate capital asset usage to a particular reporting period. Generally, three basic methods are used to allocate capital asset costs: (1) straight-line, (2) sum-of-the-years'-digits (SYD), and (3) declining-balance. These depreciation systems are a part of the asset expenditure cycle.

The transactions related to depreciation result in the following journal entries:

	Debit	Credit
Depreciation	xxxx.xx	
Asset accumulated depreciation		xxxx.xx

Here expense is increased and assets reduced through the contra-asset account of accumulated depreciation.

For Medicare reimbursement purposes, all capital assets acquired after June 1971 must be depreciated on a straight-line basis. Procedures related to straight-line depreciation allow for a constant allocation to each accounting period of the cost of the asset less any anticipated salvage value. The format for straight-line depreciation is:

$$\frac{\text{Asset cost} - \text{Salvage value}}{\text{Number of periods in asset life}} = \frac{\text{Depreciation allocation}}{\text{to each period}}$$

The SYD procedure allows for a higher allocation of costs in the early years of an asset's life and a lower allocation at the end of the asset's life cycle, as compared with straight-line. The general format for SYD depreciation for each year's computation is:

$$(\text{Asset cost} - \text{Salvage value}) \times \frac{\text{Number of years remaining in the asset's life}}{\text{Sum of the year's digits in the asset's life}} = \frac{\text{Period}}{\text{depreciation}}$$

In the declining-balance method, an allocation multiplier of twice the rate established for straight-line depreciation is usually used. This doubling of the multiplier is known as a double-declining balance. Again, a higher allocation of costs is made in the early years of the asset's life. The format for computing annual depreciation under this method is:

$$\frac{(\text{Cost of asset} - \text{Prior accumulated depreciation})}{\times (\text{Multiplier}) \times (1/\text{Asset life})} = \text{Period depreciation}$$

Note that, under this method, salvage value is not considered as a reduction of the initial cost to be depreciated. An inputted salvage value is assumed in the method, in that the balance of accumulated depreciation will never equal zero. A best estimate of salvage value may be achieved by adjustments to the multiplier.

Table 5–1 shows the computations and results for the three depreciation methods.

Depreciation policies must be formulated and approved at the highest levels of the institution. Top management must decide not only the method of computing depreciation but also when to begin depreciating the asset after it has been acquired or put into service.

Common methods of timing capitalization for depreciation are (1) month-by-month, (2) one-half year in the year of acquisition, and (3) year after acquisition.

Under month-by-month policies of capitalization, depreciation is allocated to the accounting period beginning with the month the asset is acquired or placed in service. When the asset is disposed of, depreciation allocations end with the month in which the asset is disposed of. One-half year depreciation policies allow for the allocation of depreciation for one-half year on all assets acquired during the fiscal year. One-half year depreciation is also taken for all assets in the year of their disposal. Under year-after-acquisition policies, depreciation is taken in the year after the acquisition of the asset, and a full year's depreciation is taken in the year of disposal of the asset. The most accurate procedure for timing in a depreciation policy is month-by-month; this allows for the best match of expense to the accounting period to which the asset applies.

Table 5–1 Accelerated Depreciation Methods

Sum of Years' Digits

$6000 – $600 = $5400

	1	5,400 × 10/55 =	$ 982
	2	5,400 × 9/55 =	884
	3	5,400 × 8/55 =	785
	4	5,400 × 7/55 =	687
	5	5,400 × 6/55 =	589
	6	5,400 × 5/55 =	491
	7	5,400 × 4/55 =	393
	8	5,400 × 3/55 =	295
	9	5,400 × 2/55 =	196
	10	5,400 × 1/55 =	98
Total	55		$5,400

Fixed Percentage of a Declining Balance

1	6,000 × 20%	=	$1,200
2	6,000 – 1200 = 4,800 × 20% =		960
3	6,000 – 2160 = 3,840 × 20% =		768
4	6,000 – 2928 = 3,072 × 20% =		614
5	6,000 – 3542 = 2,458 × 20% =		492

Table 5-1 continued

	6	6,000 − 4034 = 1,966 × 20% =	393
	7	6,000 − 4427 = 1,573 × 20% =	315
	8	6,000 − 4742 = 1,258 × 20% =	252
	9	6,000 − 4994 = 1,006 × 20% =	201
	10	6,000 − 5195 = 805 × 20% =	161
Total	55		$5,356

Straight-Line Depreciation

$6,000 − $600 = $5,400

	1	5,400/10 =	$540
	2	5,400/10 =	540
	3	5,400/10 =	540
	4	5,400/10 =	540
	5	5,400/10 =	540
	6	5,400/10 =	540
	7	5,400/10 =	540
	8	5,400/10 =	540
	9	5,400/10 =	540
	10	5,400/10 =	540
Total	55		$5,400

The administration must understand each of these methods so that cash flow can be maximized. The month-by-month and one-half year methods both provide higher cost reimbursement by Medicare than the year-after-acquisition method. However, ease of computation may be a factor, in which case the year-after method has the advantage.

In deciding which depreciation method to use, the administration must keep in mind several key questions:

- While Medicare reimbursement for current acquisitions is based on straight-line, which method best approximates capital usage over the life of the asset?

- What is the hospital's policy regarding funding of depreciation? If depreciation is applicable to rate setting, the recoup of asset amortization on an accelerated basis provides for advanced accumulation of funds for asset replacement.

- What are the average lives of asset categories? Overextended lives for new acquisitions result in delays in recognition of amortization and deferred Medicare reimbursement and cash flow.

The issue of asset cost allocation is related to the disposition of a capital asset. It is rare to find the actual life of an asset to be exactly equal to the original life estimated for depreciation purposes. At the end of the asset's life, any of several methods of disposition may be used: (1) sale of the asset, (2) retirement of the asset, or (3) trade-in of the asset.

As noted earlier, the recording of depreciation results in an increase in expense and a reduction in the capital asset via a contra-asset account, accumulated depreciation. In analyzing the transaction of the sale of an asset, the asset, cash, must be increased, the asset sold must be taken out of the capital asset account, the related accumulated depreciation must be eliminated for the asset, and a gain or loss must be determined on the sale of the asset. If the cash received is more than the book value (original asset cost-related accumulated depreciation), a gain is realized. Conversely, if cash received is less than the book value of the asset, a loss is realized.

Suppose a hospital sells for $6,000 in cash an asset costing $10,000 with $5,000 accumulated depreciation. The entry to record this transaction is:

	Debit	Credit
Accumulated depreciation	$5,000	
Cash	$6,000	
Capital asset		$10,000
Gain on asset disposal		$1,000

A similar analysis may be made for outright disposal of a capital asset, with the exception of the recognition of cash receipts. If the asset is not fully depreciated, the book value of the asset must be written off and a loss realized. In the above example, excluding the cash received, the entry to record the disposal of the asset would be:

	Debit	Credit
Loss on asset disposal	$5,000	
Accumulated depreciation	$5,000	
Asset		$10,000

The transaction analysis related to the trade-in of an asset begins with the disposition of the original asset, the recognition of the asset acquired at full cost, and the gain or loss realized based on the amount allowed on the trade-in and the book value of the asset disposed of. To illustrate, suppose the $10,000 asset with $5,000 accumulated depreciation was traded in on an asset costing $20,000. However, only $18,000 was paid, given the $2,000 allowance for the item traded in. The following entry is appropriate:

	Debit	Credit
Loss on asset disposal	$3,000	
Accumulated depreciation	$5,000	
Capital asset (new)	$20,000	
Cash		$18,000
Capital asset (old)		$10,000

Note the decrease in the asset, cash, and the increase in the new asset, with the difference realized as revenue per our previous analysis of revenue. However, the asset traded in had a book value that was higher than the trade-in allowance; therefore, a loss was recognized on the transaction.

While the above analysis of the trade-in of an asset details the results of the transaction, alternative methods are available to record the transaction. An example of an alternative method would be not to recognize a gain or loss. In this case, the value of the acquired asset is established at $18,000 and the old asset is kept on the books, with gains and losses recognized over the lives of the assets held on the books via increased or decreased depreciation.

Advocates of price-level depreciation, which provides for price-level adjustments to depreciation, argue that to reflect accurately the economic impact of the environment on the financial operations of the institution— basically the effects of inflation on the replacement value of assets—economic gains and losses related to the use of capital assets over an extended period of time must be taken into account. To establish a systematic method of reflecting increases in costs of replacement—which are very real—in rate structures, price-level depreciation, if used properly, may provide a valuable management tool in the accounting and reporting system. At the present time, however, generally accepted accounting principles do not recognize price-level depreciation and as a result, price-level costs are not allowed by Medicare. On this point, reasonable argument may be made that Medicare cannot continue to reimburse hospitals only on an historic cost basis without allowing rates of return or price-level adjustments for at least capital asset replacement.

Assume a $1,000 piece of equipment with a ten-year life and a policy of straight-line depreciation. As indicated in the previous discussion, annual depreciation would be $100 ($1,000 ÷ 10 = $100). The Consumer Price Index must be identified for each year of the ten-years. The conversion factor is based on the inflation factors for each year from the year of acquisition; that is, an item costing $1,000 in 1965 would cost 1.0285 times (97.2 ÷ 94.5) more in 1966 (assuming 97.2 CPI in 1966 and 94.5 in 1965), or $1,028.50.

Continuing the example, if the replacement cost in 1966 is $1,028.50, current depreciation should be $102.85 ($1,028.50 ÷ 10), and, on a retroactive basis, accumulated depreciation at the end of the second year should be $205.71 ($102.85 × 2). Therefore, the current price-level depreciation is $105.71 ($205.71 − $100.00). The normal entry to record this transaction is:

	Debit	Credit
Price-level depreciation	$5.71	
Appropriated fund balance for price-level depreciation		$5.71

Note that $100 has already been recorded for the current historic cost depreciation. Therefore, the current effect of price-level depreciation is $5.71 ($105.71 − $100.00). Also, the expense account has been increased and, to retain the integrity of historic cost accounting, an appropriation to the fund balance is made.

As noted in our discussion of other operating revenues, the matching principle requires the charging of revenues and expenses to the period in which they are earned or consumed. However, a hospital's operations do not always provide for the proper allocation of expenses at the time payment is made. An example would be a case of x-ray film received on August 15, 1979. When received, a liability is created and an expense incurred. Suppose payment is not made until September 1979. The expense must be recorded, but an asset cannot be decreased. The alternative that must be used is to increase liabilities via accounts payable. The format for the entry is:

	Debit	Credit
Expense	xxxx.xx	
Accounts payable		xxxx.xx

A similar situation exists when the end of the accounting period falls between pay dates for payroll. The usual entry for issuing pay is:

	Debit	Credit
Expense	xxxx.xx	
Cash		xxxx.xx

In this case, an accrued liability is usually established for the estimated wages earned but unpaid within an accounting period. The following case illustrates this procedure:

ABC Hospital has a biweekly pay period that began at the end of June. Four days were accrued to June, with ten days applicable to July for the pay period ending July 10. The gross pay for July 10, 1979, is $100,000. Therefore, $4 \div 14 \times \$100,000$ must be posted to June's expense, as follows:

	Debit	Credit
Departmental expense	$28,571.43	
Accrued payroll		$28,571.43

This entry must be reversed in July when actual cash is expended and posted to individual accounts. A similar method should be adopted for payroll taxes owed by the hospital, e.g., F.I.C.A., to match correctly revenues and expenses and to maximize cost reimbursement in the current period. Other examples of accrued liabilities are pension costs; interest expense; insurance expenses, including contributions to a self-insurance trust; and vested vacation earned by employees. Here, estimates of costs for the current year may be made with payments not due until a future period.

Another example of matching procedures can be seen in the case of prepaid expenses, for example, insurance premiums, leases, and rent. Here, the hospital may make payment in advance for an expenditure that benefits future time periods. The usual entry is:

	Debit	Credit
Expense	xxxx.xx	
Cash		xxxx.xx

But this does not establish proper matching. Therefore, the following entry is appropriate:

	Debit	Credit
Prepaid expense	xxxx.xx	
Expense		xxxx.xx

This entry establishes the asset that will be of benefit in the future. To illustrate, assume the hospital pays an annual premium of $10,000 for an insurance policy that is in effect from July 1, 1979, to June 30, 1980. The original entry at December 31, 1979 was:

	Debit	Credit
Insurance expense	$10,000	
Cash		$10,000

This would overstate the expense because one-half of $10,000 or $5,000.00 applies to 1980. Therefore, the adjusting journal entry to correct the situation is:

	Debit	Credit
Prepaid expense	$5,000	
Insurance expense		$5,000

A final issue related to operating expenses is the increasing use of deferred compensation by hospital-based physicians. The Internal Revenue Code provides for the deferring of compensation to future time periods for certain individuals. Generally, payments are made by the hospital for insurance policies or irrevocable trusts that will benefit the individual at some future time. Proper accounting calls for the recognition of the full expense for the services performed and the establishment of a payment mechanism for contributing to the deferred compensation instrument.

Section 5: Nonoperating Revenue

Nonoperating activities of the hospital are activities that are not within the scope of providing health care to patients. Generally, items like contributions, investment income, and gains/losses on disposal of capital items are included in this section of the statement of revenues and expenses. Since accounting procedures related to gains and/or losses on disposal of capital assets have already been described, the focus of attention here is on other areas of nonoperating income.

Contributions to hospitals, particularly contributions unrestricted as to use, have declined over the past several years. Unrestricted contributions should be reported as nonoperating income. Thus:

	Debit	Credit
Asset	xxxx.xx	
Contributions-unrestricted		xxxx.xx

Restricted contributions, discussed in Chapter 6, should be taken directly into the fund balance.

With respect to investment income, the basic procedures used to match revenues and expenses require that accruals be made throughout the year for interest earned but not received. The entry for this transaction is:

	Debit	Credit
Accrued interest receivable	xxxx.xx	
Investment income		xxxx.xx

The accrual is made by allocating total interest due from the investment based on the number of days it is held in a period compared to total days held. When the cash is received, the required entry is:

	Debit	Credit
Cash	xxxx.xx	
Accrued interest receivable		xxxx.xx
Investment income		xxxx.xx

Note that the accrual entry was reversed for the amount established as a receivable and proper period interest income was reported as revenue. As an example, suppose the hospital invests $100,000 for one year on November 30, 1979, due December 1, 1980, at 10 percent interest. Total interest is then $10,000 ($100,000 × .10 × (365 ÷ 365)). The computation for the 1979 interest receivable is:

$$\frac{\text{Number of days held in 1979}}{\text{Total number of days to be held}} = \frac{31}{365} \times \$10,000 = \$849.32$$

The entry to record this transaction is:

	Debit	Credit
Accrued interest receivable	$849.32	
Investment income		$849.32

When the investment matures, cash in the amount of $10,000 interest income will be received. The entry to record this transaction is:

	Debit	Credit
Cash	$10,000.00	
Accrued interest receivable		$849.32
Interest income		$9,150.68

The above example does not provide for monthly accruals of interest income. In practice, the accruals should be made monthly to provide the most accurate interim financial reporting.

COMMUNITY MEDICAL CENTER: COMPARATIVE ANALYSIS OF OPERATING REPORTS

An understanding of the fundamental issues related to the major categories of the statement of revenues and expenses is essential to managerial finance and accounting. Hospital administrators must be fully aware of their role in guiding the financial operations of the institution through rate setting polices, credit policies, depreciation methods, inventory pricing policies, and operational evaluation. In order to set these policies, the administrator must be familiar with the reporting procedures related to operations on both an annual and interim basis. To ensure that action is taken on a timely and meaningful basis, the administrator must be able to analyze systematically operating results not only for a particular accounting period but also on a comparative basis in relation to prior years' activities and planned (budgeted) levels of operating results.

The administrative task of financial statement analysis is extremely complex and time-consuming. The vast volumes of information available on hospital operations make it almost impossible to maintain a continuing, systematic financial review. It is therefore imperative that the hospital administration devise a system of analysis that identifies for further managerial involvement key areas of operations with the potential for increased cash flow and operational efficiencies.

At this point, the reader has available (from Chapter 2) the financial statements related to the operations of Community Medical Center for the three years 1977, 1978, and 1979. The reader should now make decisions keyed to the following managerial questions:

- How efficient have operations been in the past, and how cost-effective are they currently?

- How close have actual operations been to planned levels, and where have been the problem areas?

- What are the trends in revenue deductions? What are their sources? What causal environmental factors are at work?

- Could the medical center undertake a major expansion program at this time?

• What steps could be taken to enhance the financial operations of the institution?

To begin the analysis, the reader must decide what information to obtain, what are the objectives in using the information, and what needs to be known to manage effectively. The information important to a hospital administrator is as diverse as the objectives of an institution. There is no one, universal answer to the question, What do I need to know? There are, however, several basic guidelines that might aid in the establishment of a systematic way to analyze information related to hospital operations.

To begin with, activity data must be incorporated into the financial cycle. The reader should identify activity levels for the hospital overall and for each key operating area (Chapter 2 should be reviewed to obtain this information).

The next step is to relate activities to revenues and expenses on a per unit basis. This can usually be done on a gross basis, for example, totals per patient day. However, key operating areas can also be analyzed. In particular, the reader should perform this analysis for the areas concerned with the planned expansion project.

Based on the results of this analysis, the reader should begin to examine areas for mix of services and historic rate increases. Here, data related to the utilization of man hours are important; activity per man hours and trends in man hours are key measures of managerial efficiency. Given the salary data in previous chapters, the reader should analyze the trends in the expansion areas and determine potential efficiencies that can be achieved through altered hiring practices.

Finally, to gain the proper perspective, the reader should make a comparison of budgeted levels of activity with actual levels. Are activities on target or have rates increased beyond planned levels to cover a variance?

The reader should now be prepared to formulate some basic conclusions and decisions with respect to the five key questions posed above.

Chapter 6

The Balance Sheet

INTRODUCTION

It should be clear at this point that revenues are directly related to the increase in the value and/or volume of assets or the reduction of liabilities, resulting in a direct interfacing of the statement of revenues and expenses with assets and liabilities. The basic accounting equation, assets = liabilities + fund balance or equity, provides the structure for presenting the financial position of an institution at a given point in time. The financial statement that displays that financial position is the balance sheet. Exhibits 6–1 and 6–2 show, reproduced from Chapter 2, the balance sheets for Community Medical Center for the years 1977 and 1978, ending December 31. The key sections of the statement reflect (1) current assets; (2) property, plant, and equipment; (3) other assets; (4) current liabilities; (5) deferred revenue; (6) long-term debt; and (7) fund balance. The categorization of unrestricted and restricted funds in the balance sheet indicates the use of fund accounting principles. The reader will note that the balance sheet deals with the same areas discussed in the previous chapter relating to the statement of revenues and expenses: accumulated depreciation, inventory, accounts payable, pre-paid expenses, and reserves for uncollectable accounts.

In this chapter we will examine the format of the balance sheet and the accounting methods used in its preparation and will illustrate potential uses of this financial statement in Community Medical Center. As we progress through the seven areas of the statement, the reader should keep in mind that the information presented is more than a set of random numbers displayed in a unique format. The reader's attention should properly be focused on the meaning of the information as it reflects the important relationships involved.

Exhibit 6-1 Community Medical Center: Balance Sheet Assets for the Years 1977 and 1978 Ending December 31

Section		1978	1977
		(in 000s)	
1.	Current Assets:		
	Cash	$ 13	$ 100
	Receivables, less reserves for uncollectable accounts and contractual allowances of $995,000 and $885,000	2,941	2,508
	Inventories	297	332
	Prepaid insurance	31	15
	Total current assets	$ 3,282	$ 2,955
2.	Property, Plant, and Equipment, at cost:		
	Land	$ 579	503
	Land improvements	285	265
	Buildings and building service equipment	16,604	16,545
	Departmental equipment	2,979	2,771
	Construction in progress	553	28
		$21,000	$20,112
	Less accumulated depreciation	7,057	5,938
		$13,943	$14,174
3.	Other Assets:		
	Unamortized debt expense	$ 79	$ 96
	Board-designated funds for plant expansion:		
	Treasury bills	1,632	1,430
		$ 1,711	$ 1,526
		$18,936	$18,655
	Restricted Funds		
	Industrial Development Fund:		
	Due from unrestricted fund	$ 20	$ —
		$ 20	$ —

Exhibit 6–2 Community Medical Center: Balance Sheet Liabilities and Fund Balances for the Years 1977 and 1978 Ending December 31

Section		1978	1977
		(in 000s)	
4.	Current Liabilities:		
	Current maturities of long-term debt	$ 320	$ 295
	Note payable, 12%	10	15
	Accounts payable	910	524
	Accrued liabilities	595	595
	Other reserves	24	18
	Due to restricted fund	20	—
	Total current liabilities	$ 1,879	$ 1,447
5.	Deferred Revenues, arising from use of accelerated depreciation for Medicare and Medicaid reimbursement	$ 356	$ 340
6.	Long-Term Debt, less current maturities	$ 5,500	$ 6,000
7.	Fund Balance	$11,201	$10,868
		$18,936	$18,655
	Restricted Funds		
	Industrial Development Fund: Fund balance	$ 20	$ —
		$ 20	$ —

MAJOR SECTIONS

Section 1: Current Assets

Assets that are liquid in nature and expected to "turn over" within a relatively short period of time are classified as current assets on the balance sheet. Examples are cash, receivables (net of reserves for allowances and uncollectable accounts), inventories, and prepaid expenses. Since the basic journal entries for these assets have already been presented in the previous chapter, the discussion here will focus on the nature of these items and on the related key managerial issues.

Cash is the most liquid asset and thus provides for a great deal of flexibility in future operational use. One would generally expect that the more cash on hand, the more sound the institution. In fact, cash levels should not be more than that minimum required to maintain operations. The rationale for this relates to the alternative uses of cash and the inability of a checking account to earn interest. Given alternative investment opportunities, the soundly run institution must look for alternatives to cash holdings, such as investments in savings accounts or in operations that yield the greatest potential for a return on investment. It is imperative to determine what items make up the cash category, in order to identify whether both checking and savings accounts or short-term investments are included in the balance. Generally, cash holdings plus savings accounts are regarded as cash, due to similarities in liquidity.

Due to cash's liquidity, tight managerial control must be established for its safekeeping. In addition to the general procedures for cash control outlined in previous discussions (Chapter 3), there are some specific accounting procedures related to cash and its control. The areas involved are (1) petty cash, (2) cash collections, and (3) bank reconciliations.

Petty Cash

Daily operations of a hospital require that a certain amount of cash be disbursed for minor items, such as cab fare for an emergency delivery of supplies, parking expense while personnel attend outside seminars, registered mail, and so on. Also, a supply of change is needed for cashiering functions in the cafeteria and business office. It is almost impossible to write checks through the cash control cycle for such items; therefore, cash is held in various areas of the institution for payment of such incidental items. Several key considerations should govern the establishment of such cash funds:

- Specified areas and individuals must be authorized by the hospital's administration to maintain control of the cash in the designated areas.

- The number of areas holding cash must be limited and the amount of cash held must be only large enough to make payments of limited amounts authorized by the hospital's administration.
- Verification and authorization of the transactions must be held with the petty cash and turned into the accounting area for account distribution and replenishment of the fund.

The following accounting entries are made to establish the petty cash fund:

	Debit	Credit
Petty cash	xxxx.xx	
Regular cash		xxxx.xx

No revenue or expense is realized as a result of this transaction. Rather, one asset is increased and another asset decreased by the same amount. The following entry replenishes the fund:

	Debit	Credit
Expense	xxxx.xx	
Regular cash		xxxx.xx

The effect of this entry is to spread the disbursements made from petty cash to the proper accounts and to provide cash to replenish the fund.

Cash Collections

Specific control areas are involved in cash collection. Due to the nature of insurance payments, a significant amount of cash is collected by mail, a smaller amount is collected at the hospital from the patient, and a certain amount is collected from other areas of the institution's operations, such as interest, cafeteria, sale of capital assets, and so on. In this context, systems must be developed to ensure the following objectives:

- All cash is collected and reported.
- All cash is deposited intact in the bank on a timely basis.
- Cash receipts are properly posted to the proper general ledger account and to the proper subsidiary ledger.

Frequently the internal controls on cash delay the flows through the internal processing system. To speed processing, several hospitals are copying checks at the time of delivery to the hospital. This procedure facilitates the deposit of cash on the day it is received. Controls usually allow for independent tapes of checks and copies to ensure full information flow. Ideally, deposits made to the bank should be placed in interest-bearing instruments such as savings accounts, treasury bills, certificates of deposit, and repurchase agreements (rcpos). In an ideal situation, there is an immediate and continuous "working" of cash holdings. Only a minimal amount of cash is held in checking accounts and as idle cash; all other cash holdings are continuously working. With such cash earning a return, arrangements should be made with vendors to obtain the most extended payment terms without loss of discounts. (A further analysis of cash holdings and investments will be made in a subsequent chapter related to working capital management.)

Bank Reconciliations

A final issue related to cash and cash control concerns the reconciliation of bank statements to book balances. As noted in Chapter 3, a key element in the control of the cash control cycle is that of external verification of internally reported transactions. The volume of activity in the hospital's checking accounts and the high degree of liquidity of cash dictate continuous reconciliation of bank statements to book balances, with managerial follow-up of any identified variances. It is not uncommon for bank charges to be left unrecorded, for checks received to have insufficient funds, and for errors to appear in the bank's recording of checking account transactions. If checking transactions were instantaneously processed by the bank, with instant recording of deposits made and checks issued, theory would require that the book balance equal the bank statement. However, deposits made by the hospital that are recorded as cash increases on the hospital's books are not always recorded by the bank until one or two days after the deposit is made. Similarly, checks issued by the hospital may remain outstanding for a considerable period of time. These timing variances must be taken into account in the bank reconciliation process.

The general format for the bank reconciliation is as follows:

Balance per bank at MM/DD/YY	xxxx.xx
Deduct: Outstanding checks	(xxxx.xx)
Add: Deposits in transit	xxxx.xx
Balance per books	xxxx.xx

All cash on hand in the hospital should be reported on the balance sheet at the end of the reporting period. This should include all receipts that are on hand with the cashier at the close of the reporting period. The failure to report all cash could result in a misstatement of cash leading to inappropriate managerial decision making and action. In a similar vein, written checks should not be held for later disbursement. The practice of holding checks could result in a loss of cash control and errors in the presentation of actual liabilities at the end of the reporting period.

Many hospitals have several checking accounts designated for specific purposes. Examples are accounts for regular operations, payroll, construction, and refunds. Care should be taken to avoid interbank transfers of funds at the close of the accounting period. Such transfers could involve "kiting," where funds are continuously transferred between accounts to cover a cash shortage. Review of authorization documentation and bank statements on a detailed basis by an independent party will aid in controlling against this possibility.

Accounts Receivable

Accounts receivables constitute a substantial proportion of a hospital's liquid assets. As noted earlier, it is essential that receivables be reported on a realistic, collectable basis, that is, net of reserves for bad debts and contractual allowances. Without a realistic presentation of accounts that are likely to be collected, managerial actions of the hospital's administration may be misdirected. Beyond an understanding of the basic procedures for reserve computations as presented in the preceding chapter, the importance of receivables management and control to the fiscal viability of the institution must be emphasized. The administration of the hospital must be aware of receivables trends and procedures in line with approved credit policies.

With respect to the managerial issues related to receivables, the following key management and control points should be noted:

- Data flow into the revenue and credit systems must be timely and accurate.

- Trends in payment and carrier utilization have a direct impact on receivables; increasing utilization by cost reimbursement programs and longer periods to pay on account present a significant cause for concern regarding the viability of receivables.

- Payment cannot be expected until a bill is sent. Therefore, billings should be made on a timely and accurate basis.

- Continuous evaluation of carriers is essential to determine potential changes in coverage or processing practices.

- Information required for billing, such as discharge diagnoses, should be analyzed for potential improvement in the speed of collection and the accuracy of the data required to bill.

- Credit policies must be continuously reviewed and updated for effective action in light of current laws and environmental conditions.

- Personalized and continuous communications should be maintained with the patient. Patient involvement can help speed insurance payments. Also, in this way, the patient and hospital will both have current knowledge of the billing status and of potential problems in payment arrangements.

Receivables from other hospital operations are also recorded in the receivables section of the balance sheet. Examples include physicians' office rent, receivables from cost report settlements, and receivables from insurance claims. The managerial concerns cited above also apply to these areas.

Inventories

Inventories may be viewed as materials that have not been utilized as expense in current operations but will be utilized in future reporting periods. Generally, inventories do not account for a significant portion of a hospital's assets. However, managerial direction is still essential to properly identify areas for inventory and to determine pricing policies and physical control.

Ideally, all unused material in the facility should be subject to inventory. However, practical considerations usually limit inventory procedures to areas of significant supply volume, such as dietary, laboratory, storeroom, central supply, maintenance, operating room, housekeeping, and pharmacy. Material in areas like floor stock that have insignificant volume and are to be used only over a short period of time may not require strict inventory procedures.

Administrative input in monitoring inventory levels is essential to avoid overstocking and the carrying of obsolete goods. Such input is also needed to determine inventory pricing policy in the use of LIFO, FIFO, periodic, or perpetual procedures. To achieve efficient operations, stock should be centralized as much as possible. Control is greatly enhanced if most stock is held in areas like the storeroom or central supply. Another reason for centralization is that purchasing efficiency is directly related to the volumes of orders. Items in inventory should be reported at the lower of cost or market value, particularly in the case of obsolete items.

Prepaid Expenses

Prepaid expenses are assets that will be consumed in future direct operations of the hospital. Examples are prepaid insurance, rent, leases, and interest. Prepaid expenses are liquid to the extent that cash could be realized by the elimination of the expense; for example, cancellation of an insurance policy yields the return of the unused portion of the premium. Care must be taken to ensure the proper matching of revenues and expenses for a given period in order to provide sound and accurate managerial information. In this respect, prepaid expenses allow for the systematic allocation of expenses to future accounting periods.

Other current assets include temporary investments that are expected to be placed in operation within a relatively short period of time. The time frame here is usually one year. Such investments are generally unrestricted as to use. They are composed of relatively liquid assets, such as treasury bills, certificates of deposit, and perhaps certain longer-term savings accounts.

Section 2: Property, Plant, and Equipment

The second section of the balance sheet contains the capital assets of the hospital on a cost basis less accumulated depreciation. As noted previously, it is the responsibility of the hospital's administration to establish the basic criteria for the capitalization of an asset. Generally, items or groups of items costing over a certain dollar amount—for Medicare, $150 for one item and $300 for groups of items—with a useful life over a minimum time frame —usually one year—are the basic criteria for the capitalization of an asset. Note in Exhibit 6–1 the classification of certain expenditures as construction in progress. This area has produced significant theoretical and managerial debate as to what items should be included, when items should be placed into service, and whether or not interest on borrowed funds for construction should be included. The latter point concerns the issue of capitalization of interest.

Generally accepted accounting principles allow for either the capitalization or expensing of interest during construction. The related interest income on the construction funds are handled in a manner consistent with the method for recording interest expense. Medicare regulations require the capitalization of interest during construction. The significance of this practice is that it reduces the level of current Medicare cost reimbursement during the construction period.

Consider the following example of the Medicare treatment of interest. Assume a hospital begins a two-year construction program with 100 percent borrowing. Assume also that the following information is available:

Medicare percentage:	35%
Funds borrowed:	$10,000,000
Interest rate on borrowed funds:	10%
Annual interest:	$1,000,000
Construction period:	2 years
Construction cost:	$10,000,000
Interest income:	Year 1 = $600,000; Year 2 = $300,000

If interest is capitalized, the total cost to be depreciated after construction is $10,000,000 + ($1,000,000 × 2) − ($600,000 + $300,000) = $11,100,000. Here, interest expense is equal to zero, and there is no Medicare reimbursement during the construction period. Medicare reimbursement occurs via increased depreciation of the higher basis over the life of the asset.

If interest were expensed, the depreciation basis would be $10,000,000, the net interest expense equal to 2 × $1,000,000 − $600,000 − $300,000 = $1,100,000, and the annual increased Medicare reimbursement in the two years during construction would be as follows:

	Year 1	Year 2	Total
Interest expense	$1,000,000	$1,000,000	$2,000,000
Interest income	(600,000)	(300,000)	(900,000)
Net interest	$400,000	$700,000	$1,100,000
Medicare %	.35	.35	.35
Increased reimbursement	$140,000	$245,000	$385,000

Arguments for expensing interest during construction are based on considerations of economic equality in construction costs between equal buildings. Two buildings having the same construction costs but with one financed internally and the second financed with borrowed funds would have different bases if the interest on the second building were capitalized. Also, the argument may be advanced that the managerial decision to borrow the construction funds results in costs that should be reflected in the period of the decision. The present theory of capitalization of interest concerns the matching of revenues and expenses, in that, if the building is not in service, there is no revenue generation and the costs incurred benefit future, not current, accounting periods. The hospital administrator must be aware of these facts, particularly when a major expansion program that includes debt financing is anticipated.

Managerial issues related to capital assets that the hospital administrator should be aware of include the following:

• The capitalization limits, which must be determined by the administration, should be reasonable and in line with the general assets being acquired.

• As noted in Chapter 5, several methods of depreciation are available to the administrator: straight-line, sum-of-the-years'-digits, and declining-balance. Remember that Medicare requires straight-line depreciation for current acquisitions.

- The timing of capitalization for depreciation for one-half year, month-by-month, or year after acquisition must be decided by the hospital administration.

- Repairs that do not enhance or extend the life of the asset may be expensed.

- Asset lives that include physical deterioration and obsolescence may vary from standards. Shorter, more reasonable lives could increase cost-based reimbursement.

- Continuous comparisons of actual versus planned capital expenditures should be made at the administrative level.

A final question relating to lease arrangements is whether a lease of a capital asset is an expense or a capitalizable item. Historically, lease payments have been treated in most cases as a normal rental that was expensed. However, the Financial Accounting Standards Board has now issued Financial Accounting Standard 13 (FAS–13), which provides leasing criteria to determine whether a lease is to be treated as an operating or capital lease. Under FAS–13, if the lease meets any one of the following criteria, it is to be capitalized:

- Ownership is transferred to the lessee by the end of the lease term.

- The lease contains a bargain purchase option.

- The lease term is equal to 75 percent or more of the estimated economic life of the leased property.

- The present value at the beginning of the lease term of the minimum lease payments equals or exceeds 90 percent of the excess of the fair value of the leased property over any related investment tax credit retained by the lessor.

FAS–13 has a direct impact on accounting for the lease transaction. If the lease is determined to be a capital lease, the asset and debt are recorded at an amount equal to the present value of the lease payments, discounted at the lower of the hospital's incremental borrowing rate or the interest rate implicit in the lease. If the fair value of the leased asset at the inception of the lease is less than the discounted present value of the lease payments, the fair value becomes the amount to be recorded. The asset is then depreciated in accordance with the hospital's policy over the asset's life, or lease term if the term approximates the life of the asset. Lease payments then become debt service, with a portion debt principle retirement and the remainder interest expense. If the lease is an operating lease, there is no balance sheet effect, with the lease payment recorded as an expense.

The hospital administrator should be aware of the accounting flows related to the capital and operating leases. Under a capital lease, the capital asset is increased by the present value of the lease at the time of the incurrence of the lease, as follows:

	Debit	Credit
Capital asset	xxxx.xx	
Debt-lease		xxxx.xx

When lease payments are made, the debt is reduced for the portion of the payment applicable to the principle, and interest expense is incurred for the interest portion of the payment. The entry to record this transaction is:

	Debit	Credit
Debt-lease	xxxx.xx	
Interest expense	xxxx.xx	
Cash		xxxx.xx

Under the operating lease, no entry is required at the inception of the lease. When payments are made, the following entry is made:

	Debit	Credit
Leasing expense	xxxx.xx	
Cash		xxxx.xx

The reader should note the effects of the above transactions on the balance sheet and statement of revenues and expense.

Managerial decisions should allow for the development of the initial lease agreement that provides the best terms for the hospital. The total cash flows of the two types of leases generally are very similar. However, the accounting, recording, and reimbursement effects of the two methods may be substantially different.

Section 3: Other Assets

Assets recorded in the third section of the balance sheet include unamortized debt expense, board-designated funds for plant expansion, long-term investments, and various construction and bond-related funds.

When long-term debt is incurred, there are costs associated with the issuance of the bonds or the acquisition of the loan or mortgage, such as discounts, legal fees, and accounting fees. Generally accepted accounting principles require the amortization of these "flotation" costs over the life of the debt. Consequently, these costs must be recorded as assets at the time of payment and as expense on a prorated basis to future accounting periods on a straight-line or accelerated basis, which is usually on a percentage of the bonds outstanding. The following journal entry records unamortized debt expense:

	Debit	Credit
Unamortized debt expense	xxxx.xx	
Cash		xxxx.xx

To record the amortization of flotation costs, the following entry is made:

	Debit	Credit
Amortization of debt expense	xxxx.xx	
Unamortized debt expense		xxxx.xx

Sound financial management practice requires the accumulation of sufficient funds to replace the capital assets of the institution. The general practice in the hospital industry is to accumulate these funds via the funding of depreciation. Under this practice, amounts of cash equal to depreciation are set aside into board-designated funds for use in plant expansion and are thereby restricted for use in capital acquisitions. The funds held for such replacement are invested in interest-bearing instruments and are subject to the following managerial considerations:

- The board restriction does not allow for use of these funds for general operations.

- "Borrowing" from these funds for operations is allowable only if there is intent to provide repayment.

- Interest income on these funds does not have to be offset against allowable costs for Medicare reimbursement computations. However, interest from these funds is reported as revenue in the statement of revenues and expenses.

These considerations provide for direct administrative involvement in the development of criteria for creating funds for asset replacement.

When available funds for construction or asset replacements and enhancements are insufficient, debt may be incurred for the necessary transactions. During construction programs, funds, usually held by a trustee, are properly reported in the other-asset section of the balance sheet. In recording debt transactions, when the funds are initially established with the trustee, the following transaction is appropriate:

	Debit	Credit
Trusteed funds	xxxx.xx	
Unamortized debt expense	xxxx.xx	
Debt		xxxx.xx

Note the establishment of the other-asset category for the borrowed funds and the debt costs that are set up as unamortized debt expense. The liability is established for the debt in the amount of the full "face value" of the debt principle to be repaid.

It is essential that the hospital's administration understand the flows of the transactions related to debt and the effects of such flows on the financial position of the institution. With significant debt financing, the change in financial structures on the balance sheet can be substantial.

Section 4: Current Liabilities

The first three sections of the balance sheet related to the assets of the hospital. Our attention must now focus on the sources of the assets, that is, the liabilities and fund balances. Current liabilities are amounts to be paid by the hospital within a relatively short period of time—usually one year. Generally, this section is made up of accounts payable, notes payable, accrued liabilities, amounts due to restricted funds, current maturities of long-term debt, and amounts of service payable as a result of advance payments, such as rents received in advance. Each of these areas has already been examined. At this point, amounts due to restricted funds will be explored in greater detail in the context of fund accounting procedures.

Restricted funds are established for specific uses that are not under the discretionary control of the hospital. Funds that are generally recorded as restricted funds include pledges and endowments used only for specific construction programs and asset acquisitions and self-insurance trusts that have been established as a part of a risk-management program as an alternative to increasing malpractice insurance premiums. The reporting of these funds as restricted funds follows the formula assets = liabilities + fund balances with-in the specific funds. As an example, here is the reporting for a self-insurance fund:

Due from unrestricted funds	$ 20,000		
Self-insurance investments	180,000	Fund balance	$200,000
	$200,000		$200,000

In this example, the current liability of $20,000 is established as "due to restricted funds" to indicate the amount required to be placed in the trust from unrestricted operations, as follows:

	Debit	Credit
Insurance expense	$20,000	
Due to restricted funds		$20,000
Due from unrestricted funds	$20,000	
Self-insurance fund balance		$20,000

Note the establishment of the expense amount and the current liability. Also recorded in this entry are the restricted fund receivables from unrestricted funds and the establishment of the restricted fund balance. When the $20,000 is put into the restricted fund, the following entry is made:

	Debit	Credit
Due to restricted funds	$20,000	
Cash		$20,000

A similar analysis may be made for pledges. Assume that pledges have been received for $2,000,000 to be used only for a specific construction pro-gram. The entry to establish the restricted fund is:

	Debit	Credit
Pledges receivable	$2,000,000	
Restricted fund balance		$2,000,000

When a payment is received on a pledge, the following entry is appropriate:

	Debit	Credit
Cash	$xxx,xxx	
Due to restricted funds		$xxx,xxx
Due from unrestricted funds	$yyy,yyy	
Pledges receivable		$yyy,yyy

When an amount is expended for the restricted purpose, the following entries are made:

	Debit	Credit
Construction	$aaa,aaa	
Cash		$aaa,aaa
Restricted fund balance	$bbb,bbb	
Due from unrestricted funds		$bbb,bbb

Note the logical flow of the above entries and the potential impact on the balance sheet when substantial assets are segregated from the "normal," operational section of the statement.

The managerial importance of current liabilities stems from the fact that the amounts are due within a relatively short period of time. It is imperative that funds be made available to cover the current liabilities of the hospital. Such liquidity is a key measure of the soundness of the institution's financial position. Current assets represent the funds available to cover liabilities and are directly reflected in the definition of working capital, which is current assets minus current liabilities. The relationship of current assets, in part and in total, to current liabilities in terms of key liquidity indicators will be discussed in a later chapter.

Section 5: Deferred Revenues

In the matching of revenues, revenue deductions, and expenses with the period in which they occur, the financial statements must reflect any differences in accounting methods in the computation of third party cost settlements. The most common variance between "book" and cost reporting is in the use of accelerated depreciation for cost reporting purposes and straight-line depreciation for book purposes. As an example, suppose the hospital has straight-line depreciation of $1,000,000. However, sum-of-the-years'-digits depreciation of $1,500,000 is used for Medicare reporting purposes. Also, suppose the Medicare utilization is 50 percent. The estimated effect of using the accelerated depreciation for cost reporting purposes may be computed as follows:

Sum of the years' digits	$1,500,000
Straight line	($1,000,000)
Difference	$ 500,000
Medicare percentage	× 50%
Difference in reimbursement	$ 250,000

This analysis reveals that, by using the accelerated method for depreciation, reimbursement from Medicare is accelerated by $250,000. As noted earlier, the total depreciation taken on an asset is the same at the end of the asset's life, regardless of the depreciation method utilized. Therefore, using an accelerated method for reimbursement, during the early years of the asset's life, reimbursement will be higher; but, in the later years of the life, reimbursement will be less than straight line, so that the deferred revenue from Medicare is zero at the end of the asset's life. The entries to record the above transactions are:

	Debit	Credit
Medicare allowance (revenue deduction)	$250,000	
Deferred revenue		$250,000

Note that the above entry provides for a matching of allowances with amounts reported as revenue and expense for the current period.

Section 6: Long-Term Debt

Long-term debt may be defined as borrowings which have a life of over one year. Included would be notes, bonds, capital leases, and mortgages. All of these have terms of repayment that exceed one year.

Only the principle is reported in the long-term-debt section of the balance sheet. Future interest payments due are recorded as accrued liabilities during the time period to which they relate and are at that point expensed. Any current maturity of long-term debt principle should be reported as a current liability and as a contra-item reducing the balance of the long-term debt section.

Long-term financing may take several forms, each of which must be analyzed in depth by the hospital administration to ascertain the most beneficial terms in light of the hospital's particular circumstances. The most common types of financing instruments are (1) capital leases, (2) mortgages, (3) taxable bonds, (4) tax-exempt bonds, and (5) notes payable.

Capital Leases

As we have noted, leases have many of the same components as debt and, in increasing numbers of instances since FAS–13 was issued, are recorded in the same format as debt. Generally, the format of a lease agreement contains a description of the asset and a required payment pattern—usually monthly—for the term of the lease. Inputted in the payment schedule is a charge for financing, interest, and in some cases maintenance agreement payments.

Even in a not-for-profit institution, which is exempt from sales tax, the lessee under a lease arrangement is usually responsible for payment of sales tax, in that title does not pass to the lessee from the lessor for at least the life of the lease. The hospital should exercise extreme care in assessing the full import of the lease agreement before a commitment is made. Lease terms may appear initially attractive and arrangements made quickly, only to discover that the terms are severely restrictive in practice.

Mortgages

A second source of financing available to a hospital is a loan secured by the hospital's property via a mortgage arrangement. Mortgage arrangements may be made with several sources of funds—banks, insurance companies, and so on—and are usually for a term of 10 to 15 years. Front-end costs are usually small, approximating 1 to 2 percent of the amount financed. Interest rates are usually at the upper end of the range of general bond rates. Payments are generally made at the completion of the project, necessitating interim financing during construction. Usually, mortgage terms are "closed-end" financings, in that additional borrowing is precluded by the mortgage. In most instances, about 50 to 60 percent of the project cost is financed. This requires a heavy participation by the hospital. Finally, prepayment of the mortgage is restricted to ensure continued interest arrangements and to preclude refinancing at a lower rate of interest. This provision ensures a stable cash flow to the lender for the term of the mortgage.

Taxable Bonds

Another source of funds for hospital projects are bonds sold to the general public. Here, interest paid by the hospital is taxable to the bond holder. The basic components of a normal sale of bonds include the following flows:

- An investment banker or underwriter is hired to "float" the issue.

- Terms of the sale are agreed to by the hospital and the underwriter via the bond indenture and mortgage.

- A trustee is selected and agreed to by the hospital and underwriter. The trustee acts on the behalf of the bond holders.

- A sales agreement is negotiated with the investment banker. The underwriting may be "firm" or "best efforts." In a firm underwriting situation, the underwriter guarantees that the bonds will be sold, and the hospital receives a check for the selling price of the bonds less the underwriting fee at the completion of the sales agreement. In a best-efforts underwriting, the hospital receives its funds only as the bonds are sold, which substantially increases the risk to the hospital, compared with a firm underwriting.

- Bonds are printed, endorsed, and sold at par, premium, or discount.

Bond rates are dependent on market conditions and on the grade of risk of the bonds as determined by a rating agency such as Moodys, Standard and Poors, or Fitch. The normal life of the bond is 20 years, and the average flotation costs are 2 to 3 percent of the issue. Financing may be made through taxable bonds for up to about 80 percent of the project's costs. Funds can be received "front-end," eliminating the need for interim financing during construction. Bonds are generally open-end financings, in that additional debt may be incurred (usually a minimum financial position is required before the added debt is allowed). Refinancing and prepayment are usually allowed after a minimum period of time, normally 5 years.

Tax-Exempt Bonds

The issuance of tax-exempt bonds is similar to that for taxable bonds, with the exception that the interest payments for the bond holder are exempt from federal income taxes. Some states do not allow the issuing of tax exempt bonds by private institutions. However, an increasing number of states now permit this through "home rule" provisions in the state's constitution.

The bonds must be issued by a municipality or state agency to achieve tax-exempt status. Historically, title to the property passed to the municipality when the bonds were retired. However, home rule allows for a "pass-through" mortgage where the bonds are issued in the name of the municipality and are serviced by revenues of the hospital. Here, title remains with the hospital, and there is no obligation of the municipality to guarantee the bonds. As tax-exempt bonds, their interest rates are usually two to three percent lower than those of other financing instruments.

Generally, the terms of the bonds allow for open-ended future financing and for prepayment after a minimum waiting period. Usually, the term of the bonds is about 30 years, with almost total financing available at the beginning of the project, thus eliminating the need for interim financing. There are, however, several costs associated with tax-exempt financing that increase the amount of the borrowing, for example, higher front-end flotation costs such as legal fees, feasibility studies, and underwriting discounts of two to three percent.

Notes Payable

A fifth alternative is notes payable, which represent secured or unsecured borrowings from banks, individuals, savings and loans institutions, and so on.

The notes are for relatively short periods of time and for limited amounts. Promissory notes are useful in the establishment of terms for debt acquisition in cases where limited funds are needed over a relatively short period of time, such as during construction. Interest rates are usually tied to the prime or bank rate for debt and fluctuate over a relatively wide range.

In summary, when the hospital administrator evaluates potential debt in the context of the hospital's financial statements, the potential impacts of each method of debt incurrence must be carefully evaluated to determine the most favorable terms for the hospital.

Section 7: Fund Balance

The general fund balance represents the equity section of the balance sheet. Excesses and deficiencies of revenues versus expenses from the statement of revenues and expenses are recorded in this section. The flow from the statement of revenues and expenses to the fund balance "closes" the revenue and expense accounts from operations as reflected in the financial position of the institution. An expanded format for the accounting equation assets = liabilities + fund balance to reflect these flows would be $assets_t$ = $liabilities_t$ + fund $balance_{t-1}$ + net $income_t$, where t is the current period and t − 1 is the previous period.

Besides "capturing" the results of operations, this section of the balance sheet includes restricted contributions. The rationale for this practice stems from the description of the statement of revenues and expenses as a statement that reports the results of operations for a particular period. Restricted contributions may be viewed as unrelated to operations, but they do increase the assets of the institution and the fund balance. At the present time, Medicare has taken a similar position, in that restricted contributions do not have to be offset against allowable costs.

Finally, because accumulated price-level depreciation reduces the funds available for future plant acquisitions, the fund balance must be reduced by the amount of the reduced replacement capacity. To achieve this, a reduction is made in the fund balance to show the potential impact of inflation on the replacement of consumed capital assets.

SUMMARY

In analyzing the flow of transactions through the balance sheet, the hospital administrator should become familiar with the individual elements of the statement and how they interrelate with the financial operations of the institution.

At this point, the reader should be able to identify key trends in the financial position of the institution—for example, liquidity in the relation of current assets to current liabilities, debt as related to assets, fund balances known as leverage, trends in receivables and capital assets, and so on. Given this background, our focus will now shift to Community Medical Center and to the key factors in the balance sheet related to managerial decision making.

COMMUNITY MEDICAL CENTER: BALANCE SHEET

Questions that were raised earlier in our review of the statements of revenue and expense for Community Medical Center related to the soundness of the center's operations over several fiscal years and to its potential operating performance in the future. At this point, the reader should be able to address systematically the key issues in the center's financial position as presented in its balance sheets for the years 1977 to 1979. These statements are reproduced from Chapter 2 as Exhibits 6–3 and 6–4.

Exhibit 6–3 Community Medical Center: Balance Sheet Assets, for the Years 1978 and 1979 Ending December 31

	1979	1978
	(in 000s)	
Current Assets:		
Cash	$ 3	$ 13
Receivables, less reserves for uncollectable accounts and contractual allowances of $824,000 and $995,000	3,273	2,941
Inventories	320	297
Prepaid insurance	32	31
Total current assets	$ 3,628	$ 3,282
Property, Plant, and Equipment, at cost:		
Land	$ 779	$ 579
Land improvements	297	285

Exhibit 6–3 continued

Buildings and building service equipment	16,932	16,604
Departmental equipment	3,426	2,979
Construction in progress	1,411	553
	$22,845	$21,000
Less accumulated depreciation	8,126	7,057
	$14,719	$13,943
Other Assets:		
Unamortized debt expense	$ 63	$ 79
Board-designated funds for plant expansion:		
Certificates of deposit	1,026	1,632
	$ 1,089	$ 1,711
	$19,436	$18,936
Restricted Funds:		
Industrial Development Fund:		
Due from unrestricted fund	$ —	$ 20

Exhibit 6–4 Community Medical Center: Balance Sheet Liabilities and Fund Balance for the Years 1978 and 1979 Ending December 31

	1979	1978
	(in 000s)	
Current Liabilities:		
Short-term bank loan, 12%	$ 150	$ —
Current maturities of long-term debt	347	320
Notes payable	95	10
Accounts payable	964	910
Accrued liabilities	674	595
Other reserves	24	24
Due to restricted fund	—	20
Total current liabilities	$ 2,254	$ 1,879

Exhibit 6–4 continued

Deferred Revenues, arising from use of accelerated depreciation for Medicare reimbursement	$ 366	$ 356
Long-Term Debt, less current maturities	$ 5,180	$ 5,500
Fund Balance	$11,636	$11,201
	$19,436	$18,936
Restricted Fund: Industrial Development Fund: Fund balance	$ —	$ 20

The following key issues should be addressed in the analysis of Community Medical Center's balance sheets:

- What is the ability of the center to provide for adequate liquidity? How do current assets relate to current liabilities?

- What proportion of assets is financed by debt?

- What are the trends in accounts receivable balances related to charge increases?

- To what extent has depreciation been funded, and what has been the growth in investments related to operations?

- What is the ability of the center to finance an expansion program?

- What are the indications for flexibility in financing future operations?

- What is the level of capitalization of the institution—the proportion of total assets that is classified as capital assets?

In addition, as president of Community Medical Center, the reader should be able to identify potentially unfavorable trends in the financial position of the center.

Chapter 7

Supporting Schedules

INTRODUCTION

A systematic approach to analyzing the financial operations and position of the institution requires a detailed reformulation of the previously discussed financial statements. While adequate information is available in the balance sheet and statement of revenues and expenses the user may be interested in specific areas and changes in the statements. Consequently, in general practice, supporting schedules for alternative analyses have been developed. Examples are (1) the statement of change in financial position (working capital), (2) the statement of cash flow, (3) the statement of change in fund balances, and (4) other managerial schedules that detail various aspects of revenues, expenses, and other operating and nonoperating items. The analysis and development format for these schedules are indicative of a useful managerial process. Additional schedules may be developed as particular issues are identified.

The following discussion will identify the development and use of the schedules and the key managerial issues related to their function.

STATEMENT OF CHANGE IN FINANCIAL POSITION

The statement of change in financial position (working capital) shows the flow of funds related to the change between periods of the working capital (current assets − current liabilities) of the institution. Exhibit 7–1 shows this statement for Community Medical Center for 1977 and 1978, as reproduced from Chapter 2. Note the flows of assets and changes in liabilities in the statement. Both income and nonworking capital expenditures—for example, depreciation and amortization of debt expense—are sources of funds. Applications of funds relate to increases in noncurrent assets or reductions in noncurrent liabilities. Similarly, decreases in noncurrent assets and increases in liabilities are sources of working capital. The last section of the statement proves the change computed in the upper section, illustrating the change in the components of working capital. The reader should refer to the center's balance sheets and statements of revenue and expense to follow the flows into the statement of change in financial position.

Exhibit 7–1 Community Medical Center: Statements of Changes in Financial Position of Unrestricted Funds for the Years 1977 and 1978 Ending December 31

	1978	1977
	(in 000s)	
Sources of Funds:		
Operations:		
Income (loss) from operations	$ 113	$ 416
Noncash charges against income:		
Provision for depreciation-cost	1,119	1,139
Amortization of debt expense	17	20
Increase in deferred revenues	16	33
Funds provided from operations	1,265	1,608
Contributions and interest income	164	158
Transfer from Industrial Development Fund to finance property and equipment additions	56	137
	$1,485	$1,903
Applications of Funds:		
Additions to property and equipment, net	888	507
Increase in board-designated funds for plant expansion	202	608

Exhibit 7-1 continued

Reduction of long-term debt	500	300
	$1,590	$1,415
Increase (Decrease) in Working Capital	$ (105)	$ 488
Changes in Components of Working Capital:		
Current assets, increase (decrease):		
Cash	$ (87)	(40)
Receivables	433	952
Inventories	(35)	50
Prepaid insurance	16	(5)
	$ 327	957
Current liabilities, increase (decrease):		
Current maturities of long-term debt	$ 25	$ 9
Notes payable to banks and other	(5)	(5)
Accounts payable	386	224
Accrued liabilities	—	240
Specific purpose reserve	6	1
Due to restricted fund	20	—
	$ 432	$ 469
Increased (Decrease) in Working Capital	$ (105)	$ 488

The primary purpose of the latter statement is to illustrate the reasons for an increase or decrease in working capital between reporting periods. The statement provides a composite view of how financial operations have impacted the financial position of the institution. A comparison of the changes in working capital over time provides a detailed management tool that is useful in analyzing the fund flows and in identifying key trends that may require managerial intervention. The important issues and relationships in the statement are the following:

• How does funding depreciation compare to administrative goals?

- Is the center utilizing increases in liabilities significantly to fund working capital?

- Within the change in working capital components, how has cash performed over time?

- Are assets liquid enough to provide adequate coverage for current liabilities?

- Is the center maintaining the financial plan of the institution through working capital management?

- Is the ability of the center to generate increases in working capital sufficient to service debt and/or expenditures related to a major expansion program?

STATEMENT OF CASH FLOW

As noted earlier, several major considerations relate to the absolute liquidity of a hospital. Therefore, an extension of the statement of change in financial position to a statement of cash flow is appropriate. Exhibit 7–2 shows the statements of cash flow for 1977 and 1978 for Community Medical Center. The development of the statement is the same as for the statement of change in financial position, with increases in noncash assets as uses of funds and increases in liabilities and fund balances as sources of funds. Note the flows from the statement of revenue and expense and balance sheet through the statement of cash flow. With regard to this statement, the key issues and relationships of importance are:

- What are the trends in receivables and what proportions of working capital are related to changes in receivables balances?

- Are cash balances adequately invested in interest-bearing instruments?

- Do inventory build-ups appear excessive?

- Is cash flow in line with managerial plans?

- What is the ability of the center to contain cash uses and to increase cash sources?

- What is the importance of noncash flow expenses in the generation of cash flow?

Exhibit 7-2 Community Medical Center: Statements of Cash Flows for the Years 1977 and 1978 Ending December 31

	1978	1977
Sources of Funds:		
Operations:		
Income (loss) from operations	$(218,722)	$187,346
Noncash charges against income:		
Cost depreciation	1,124,877	1,138,814
Price level depreciation	330,856	228,693
Amortization of debt	17,649	19,669
Increase in deferred revenue	16,095	33,024
Funds from operations	1,270,755	1,607,546
Contributions and interest income	164,714	157,512
Transfer from Industrial Development Fund	56,026	137,503
Increase in current maturity	25,000	9,265
Increase in accounts payable	385,683	163,223
Increase in accrued liabilities	(862)	239,895
Medicare current financing advance	—	(53,400)
Specific purpose reserve	5,937	909
Total Sources of Funds	1,907,253	2,262,453
Applications of Funds:		
Cumulative effect of change in vacation pay		102,086
Net additions to property	894,030	506,963
Increase in funded depreciation	375,000	607,685
Reduction in long-term debt	326,000	313,100
Increase in receivables	433,318	723,147
Decrease in notes payable	5,000	5,000
Due to restricted fund	(20,000)	—
Increase in inventories	(35,072)	49,729
Increase in prepaid insurance	15,548	(4,727)
Total Uses of Funds	$1,993,824	$2,302,983
Increase (Decrease) in Cash	$ (86,571)	$ (40,530)

In addition to the aggregate, hospital-wide statement of cash flow, it is possible to develop cash flow statements for specific areas of the hospital's existing or planned operations. The general format for these statements is illustrated in Exhibit 7–3.

This format allows for an individualized, departmental cash flow statement for each revenue center. Its advantages lie in the ability of management to deduce from it the adequacy of charging policies by area, the impact of potential cost savings, and the adherence to cost containment activities in accordance with administrative guidelines.

Exhibit 7–3 Format for Statement of Cash Flow

Gross Revenue	$xxx,xxx
Direct Expense	(xxx,xxx)
Indirect Expense Allocation	(xxx,xxx)
Depreciation	(xxx,xxx)
Other Operating Revenue	xxx,xxx
Net Operating Income Before Revenue Deductions	$yyy,yyy
Cost Reimbursement Percentage	× .zzz
Contractual Allowances	$aaa,aaa
Net Operating Income Before Revenue Deductions	$yyy,yyy
Contractual Allowances	(aaa,aaa)
Bad Debts (gross revenue × percentage)	(ccc,ccc)
Depreciation	xxx,xxx
Change in Other Balance Sheet Categories	ddd,ddd
Cash Flow	$rrr,rrr

Potential sources of the information required in the statement of cash flow include:

- Gross revenue: General ledger of departmental revenue summaries.

- Direct expense: General ledger detail or departmental expense summary records.

- Depreciation: From a cost allocation; the Medicare cost report may be used for general information.

- Other operating revenue: Allocation of other operating revenue based on the relationship of (departmental revenue − direct expense) to (total revenue − direct expense of revenue-producing departments).

- Bad debts: Allocation of bad debts as a percentage of departmental revenue.

- Indirect expense: From a cost allocation derived in general from the Medicare cost report.

- Contractual allowances: Based on actual cost report computations of gross revenue for Medicare and Medicaid; on reimbursable costs of these programs on a departmental basis.

- Change in other cash flow items: Items such as the change in accounts receivable, debt, payables, and capital acquisitions could be allocated based on net departmental operating results (gross revenue − direct expense − indirect expense + nonoperating revenue − revenue deductions + depreciation). Direct allocation of departmental capital additions should be utilized if available.

As can be seen, the task of determining departmental cash flows is extremely complex. Additional difficulties arise when interdepartmental interactions are incorporated, for example, central supply services allocated to operating room based on requisitions for surgical packs and sterilization of instruments.

To illustrate the above points, an example of a laboratory cash flow analysis for Community Medical Center is presented in Exhibit 7–4.

A critical analysis of the Exhibit 7–4 cash flow statement reveals several interesting areas. First, a more direct allocation of depreciation may be available via a departmental analysis of capital outlays rather than by using the cost report computation. This could also apply to other indirect expenses for which alternative allocation methods may provide a more rational allocation of full cost rather than adjusted cost from the cost report. It is also possible that a more rational method could be found to allocate other revenues to a particular department. However, it may be argued that direct revenues less expenses provide at least an indication of the profitability of the area from which funds flow to perform other functions.

Exhibit 7-4 Community Medical Center: Laboratory Cash Flow Analysis for 1978 Including Price-Level Depreciation

Gross Revenue		$1,985,369
Direct Expense		$ 684,890
Depreciation		$ 36,885
Other Indirect Expense:		
Medicare Cost Report	$ 1,010,979	
Direct expense	(684,890)	
Depreciation	(36,885)	$ 289,204
Bad Debts:		
Total bad debts	$ 783,275	
Gross revenue	+ $15,970,794	
Bad debt percentage	4.90%	
Laboratory gross revenue	$ 1,985,369	
	× .0490	$ 97,283

Other Revenue:

Total other revenue	$ 386,684	

$$\frac{\text{Laboratory gross revenue} - \text{Laboratory Direct Expense}}{\text{Total gross revenue} - \text{Direct expense}} =$$

($1,985,369 − $684,890)/($15,970,794 − $5,583,887) =

.1252 ; .1252 × $386,684 =		$48,414

Contractual Allowances:

Medicare:		
Gross Medicare lab revenue	$603,089	
Medicare expense	(297,199)	
Inpatient	(1,928)	
Outpatient	(10,751)	$293,211
Medicare (computed as above)		$191,175

Other Cash Flow Items (allocated as a percentage of cash flows):

Amortization of debt	$17,649
Increase in deferred revenues	16,095
Transfer from plant replacement	56,026

Exhibit 7–4 continued

Additions to property	(894,030)
Increase in board-designated funds	(375,000)
Reduction of long-term debt	(326,000)
Increase in receivables	(433,318)
Reduction in inventories	35,072
Increase in prepaids	(15,548)
Increase in current maturities	25,000
Reduction in notes payable	(5,000)
Increase in accounts payable	385,683
Decrease in accrued liabilities	(862)
Due to restricted fund	20,000
Specific purpose reserve	5,937
Net, other cash flow items	(1,488,296)

Laboratory Cash Flows:
Gross revenue − Direct expense − Indirect expense + Nonoperating revenue − Revenue deductions + Depreciation =
$1,985,369 − $684,890 − $289,204 + $48,414 − ($97,283 + $293,211 + $191,175) = $478,020 (gross cash flows)
(Note: Depreciation is not included in other indirect expenses)

Overall Cash Flows (allocation of other cash flow items):

Overall Net Income	($54,008)
Depreciation:	
Cost	1,124,877
Price level	330,856
	$1,401,725

$478,020 ÷ $1,401,725 = .3410
($1,488,296) × .3410 = ($507,543)
Therefore, the laboratory cash flow for 1978 is ($29,523).

Direct allocations for other revenue items should be made as often as possible. It is imperative that full financial operations and cash flow be reflected in the departmental cash flow statement. This includes financial operations and practices that are not directly reflected in the statement of revenues and expenses, for example, changes in receivables, capital acquisitions, and so forth. Again, while a direct allocation of inventory changes and capital acquisitions enhances the identification of cash flow, it is reasonable to allocate other cash flow items on the basis of direct departmental "profitability."

The reader should be aware at this point that, from a cash flow standpoint, increases in noncash assets are a use of cash while increases in liabilities are a source of cash. This is intuitively reasonable and thus adds a further dimension to the analysis of the institution's fiscal operations. The administrator must be concerned not only with revenues and expenses but also with the importance for financial management of utilizing "balance sheet management" to enhance the institution's cash liquidity.

The above departmental analysis is a complete cash analysis for the operations of the department over a period of time. A similar analysis may be developed for individual segments of a revenue department and for anticipated changes in operations. In focusing on anticipated alterations to existing operations, such as adding or deleting services, it is essential to identify incremental cash items associated with the service being evaluated. Incremental cash items that would be affected by altering operations include at least the following:

- revenues from the service

- direct expenses increased or reduced by the service

- indirect expenses that would be added or deleted

- bad debts and contractual allowances that would change as a result of altering operations

- capital items required for the service

- incremental additions to other cash flow items

To illustrate, suppose the hospital is evaluating the purchase of a $500,000 piece of x-ray equipment to perform tests that to date have not been performed, that is, there would be no reduction in existing procedures. An analysis of cash flows related to this decision would be concerned with the following questions:

- What costs are to be incurred or reduced?

- Will additional revenue be generated?

- What is the life of the equipment and/or renovation?

- What is the cost reimbursement effect?

- What is the effect on indirect costs?

- What terms of equipment payment may be negotiated? Monthly installments, rentals, leases, or debt?

- What is the quality of tests performed by the equipment compared to manual procedures?

- Are there alternative sources for the performance of the anticipated procedure, for example, other hospitals, outside labs?

- Are there carry-over effects to other areas, such as exclusion of present tests or reduced patient stays?

- What is the status of the medical staff's support of the program, equipment, and procedures?

- What charge is to be made, and what is the market for the tests, such as present patients, other hospitals, new patients?

The data collection and investigative efforts to answer the above questions will be discussed at a later point. Here, we are concerned with the format for the cash flow statement related to the purchase of the x-ray equipment. The basic data related to the equipment are presented as follows.

Receivables: 70 days to pay
Equipment cost: $100,000 payable at delivery
Utilization: three procedures per day from existing patients
       : ten patients per month additional due to machine
        (the average length of stay for these additional patients is three days)
       : 30 procedures per year from other hospitals
Charge per procedure: customary charge per procedure is $100
Cost payer utilization: 45%
Cash costs to be incurred: $70,000 per year
Equipment life: ten years with no salvage value
Bad debts: 5%

The statement of projected cash flow related to the purchase of the equipment is as follows.

Revenue: (1245 procedures @ $100) + (10 × 3 × $200
      additional) $196,500

Direct Expense: $70,000 from procedures + $57,600 from added patients	− 127,600
Depreciation: $100,000/10	− 10,000
	$ 58,900
Cost Reimbursement Percentage	.45
Contractual Allowances	$ 26,505
Increase in Receivables: ($196,500/365) × 70	$ 37,685
Bad Debts: $196,500 × .05	$ 9,825
First Year Cash Flow:	
Equipment cost	($100,000)
Revenue	196,500
Direct expense	(127,600)
Contractual allowances	(26,505)
Bad debts	(9,825)
Increase in receivables	(37,685)
Cash Flow	($105,115)
Second to tenth year cash flow:	
Revenue	$196,500
Direct expense	(127,600)
Contractual allowances	(26,505)
Bad debts	(9,825)
Cash Flow	$ 32,570
Eleventh Year Cash Flow:	
Decrease in Receivables	$ 37,685

The increase in receivables is computed on a gross charge basis, based on the average numbers of days revenue in receivables. If the hospital is on PIP payments from Medicare, it may be argued that the increase in receivables should be computed on a net charge to private pay, less a reserve for bad debts. In any case, the timing differences in cash flow due to receipts of payments must be reflected in the statement of cash flow. In the above example, if the average days to pay is 70 in the first year, a lag of 70 × the average daily charge will be the increase in receivables. Assuming no change in days to pay, there will be no change in receivables until the end of the project's life, when receivables will be reduced by the 70 × average daily charge.

Any additional cash flow items, such as increases in accounts payable if appropriate to the overall analysis, would have to be included in the analysis. However, any increases in other areas may be offset by increases in various areas of the balance sheet.

At this point, a generalized format for the computation of cash flow may be developed. For ease of computation we will use the following abbreviations:

Gross revenue	GR
Expenses	E
Cost reimbursement %	CR%

Days to pay	DP
Depreciation	DEPR
Bad Debt %	BD%

From our previous discussion, we have the following equation:

$$\text{Cash Flow} = (GR - E) - CR\%(GR - E - DEPR) - BD\%(GR) - GR(DP \div 365)$$

Combining similar terms, we have:

$$
\begin{aligned}
\text{Cash Flow} &= GR - E - (CR\% \times GR) + (CR\% \times E) + (CR\% \times DEPR) - (BD\% \times \\
&\quad GR) - GR(DP \div 365) \\
&= GR - (CR\% \times GR) - (BD\% \times GR) - GR(DP \div 365) - E + (CR\% \times \\
&\quad E) + (CR\% \times DEPR) \\
&= GR(1 - CR\% - BD\% - DP/365) - E(1 - CR\%) + (CR\% \times DEPR).
\end{aligned}
$$

Note how the format of this equation relates to the contractual allowance estimation procedure described in Chapter 4. In this context, the reader should recognize the direct impact of revenue deductions, receivable increases, and depreciation on the cash flow of the project. As an exercise, the reader should test the above formula on the data of the laboratory case discussed previously. It cannot be overemphasized that the impact of revenue deductions, bad debts, and increases in receivables is substantial. This fact is readily apparent in the first section of the derived formula.

STATEMENT OF CHANGE IN FUND BALANCE

The statement of change in fund balances shows what changes have occurred in this section of the balance sheet. The statements of change in fund balance for Community Medical Center for the years 1977 and 1978 ending December 31 are reproduced from Chapter 2 as Exhibit 7–5. Note the flows of funds from the statement of revenues and expenses into the unrestricted fund balance, including price level depreciation, which is an appropriation of the fund balance. Note also the flows when funds restricted as to use are placed into operations. For 1978, $76,000 was received as restricted contributions, with $56,000 placed into operations, leaving a balance of $20,000 in restricted funds.

The statement of change in fund balance relates to the full disclosure of fund flows in the equity or fund balance sections of the balance sheet. Without such a statement, interfund transfers, appropriated funds, and other effects such as prior year changes would not be disclosed. From a managerial viewpoint, this statement is useful to identify restricted fund activities and to determine the overall impact on financial operations of such activities as a capital acquisition fund drive, donations for specific purposes, and other restricted fund activities.

Exhibit 7–5 Community Medical Center: Statements of Changes in Fund Balances, for the Years 1977 and 1978 Ending December 31

	1978	1977
	(in 000s)	
Unrestricted Funds		
Balance Beginning of Year	$10,868	$10,157
Add (Deduct):		
Excess (deficiency) of revenues over expenses	277	574
Transfer from plant replacement fund to finance property and equipment additions	56	137
Balance End of Year	$11,201	$10,868
Restricted Funds		
Industrial Development Fund:		
Balance Beginning of Year	$ —	$ 44
Add (Deduct):		
Grants	—	93
Pledge write-offs	—	(24)
Contributions	76	24
Transfer to unrestricted funds	(56)	(137)
Balance End of Year	$ 20	$ —

It is increasingly important that hospitals actively seek to develop all contribution sources. As cost reimbursement and containment activities reduce the income-generating potential of the health care institution, such drives will become increasingly important in the future of the hospital. Furthermore, community support as evidenced by a giving program is a direct benefit when dealing with external agencies, such as bond rating agencies, that identify the status of the hospital in the community.

OTHER SCHEDULES OF OPERATION COMPONENTS

It is important that the hospital's administration be directly involved in the development of all informational flows of data that are necessary as inputs into the decision-making process. Detail for any single year is useful only if compared with some base, for example, budget or prior year operations.

Under the theory of management by exception, managerial involvement is directed to those areas experiencing significant variances from budgeted levels of operations. In determining where such attention should be focused, dollar as well as percentage variances are important.

COMMUNITY MEDICAL CENTER: PRELIMINARY ANALYSIS OF EXPANSION PROGRAM

The reader should now consider the following items and questions regarding the planned expansion program at Community Medical Center as outlined in Chapter 2:

- Scope: Construction of an off-site psychiatric facility, expansion of radiology, emergency room, and laboratory areas, a new power plant, expansion of medical records and physicians' lounge, expansion of cafeteria space, and a multilevel parking garage.

- Cost: Total construction and equipment costs are estimated to be $20 million.

- Some type of long-term debt is assumed to be the most viable means of financing.

- Assuming a minimum debt package of about $25 million, including the refinancing of existing debt, what impact on the medical center's financial position do you envision?

- With regard to the statistical trends presented in Chapter 2, do you foresee growth in the utilization of the institution?

- If debt service is set at $2 million per year, depreciation over 17 years is on a straight-line basis, and cost reimbursement utilization is 50 percent, what effects would you expect on the center's cash flow?

Part III

Managerial Issues in Hospital Finance: The Action Phase

Previous sections have dealt with general financial and environmental factors in hospital management. The purpose of the present section is to identify key managerial techniques and issues that are essential to the sound administration of the institution. The organization of this part is structured on a foundation of specific techniques of financial analysis and management with application to the current hospital's environmental issues. The reader should focus on the specific methods presented and identify points that are applicable to the general case.

Chapter 8 examines ratio analysis and its applicability to hospital financial management and financial analysis. The strengths and weaknesses of ratio comparisons will be discussed. Further application of ratio analysis will be made to financial planning models and administrative decision points in setting fundamental goals and objectives.

Chapter 9 discusses working capital management. The emphasis on liquidity in the current hospital environment and the ability of the hospital's administration to impact working capital significantly via policies and procedures that control cash, investments, receivables, inventory, payables, and short-term debt necessitates a detailed review and analysis of the components of working capital (current assets — current liabilities). The management of insurance coverages and coinsurance falls indirectly within the working capital management framework. The individual components of working capital are discussed, and the key issues related to management are illustrated in the case of Community Medical Center.

A critical issue affecting hospitals is that of maximizing third party cost reimbursement, particularly Medicare. Having reviewed the basics of the Medicare program in Chapter 4, the reader is now in a position to analyze in Chapter 10 current practices to deal more effectively with the Medicare program. Topics covered in Chapter 10 include rate analysis to maximize reimbursement, analysis of cost centers that may be separately reported, analysis of cost to charge and utilization percentages in reimbursement, and the Medicare appeal process.

Chapter 11 deals with capital asset evaluation and the techniques useful in analyzing capital asset acquisitions. The current emphasis on capital asset and program evaluation mandated by P.L. 93–641, which established the local Health Systems Agencies (HSAs), and state certificate-of-need legislation requires the development of a systematic and comprehensive approach to capital asset evaluation. The several methods discussed in this chapter include payback, rate of return, and present value analysis. The pros and cons of each method are evaluated and illustrated via the case hospital, for which key managerial information and data are outlined. This is followed by an analysis of lease versus buy decisions.

Long-term financing has become increasingly important in the hospital field. Historic cost reimbursement, inflation, and a general lack of funds generation have lead to the necessity of debt financing of asset acquisitions. Furthermore, the reduced level of philanthropy has led to the use of leverage (which involves the level of debt related to assets) via debt in asset financing. Chapter 11 discusses leverage as it relates to alternative vehicles of long-term debt financing. Also, mortgage financing, taxable bonds, and tax-exempt bonds are examined as instruments of long-term debt. Comparisons of each approach are made, utilizing the techniques presented previously.

The final chapter in this section, Chapter 12, discusses current environmental factors that are having a direct impact on the financial operations of the hospital. Specifically, IRS regulations and reporting, risk management and self-insurance programs, and the proposed system for hospital uniform reporting (SHUR), currently the annual hospital report (AHR), are discussed in general terms, tying managerial issues into the direct operations of the case of Community Medical Center.

Ratio Analysis

INTRODUCTION

Previous chapters have emphasized managerial analysis and decision making relative to the financial position and operations of the hospital. As we begin a discussion of managerial action strategy, a framework must be established to allow for the identification of financial interrelationships on a comparable basis with internal and external operations and relations. A useful tool in analyzing financial operations and current financial positions is ratio analysis. The concept of ratio analysis is intuitively appealing, in that one must identify the ways in which segments of financial operations relate to each other. Previous discussions of the balance sheet and statement of revenues and expenses were based on an informal, judgmental type of analysis. In the present chapter, we begin the formulation of a systematic analytical framework based on the concept of ratio analysis. In applying ratio analysis, care must be taken to use it on consistent data and as only one input into decision making.

Ratio analysis is the comparison of segments of the financial statements with each other in a systematic way, based in at least five identifiable operating areas: liquidity, leverage, composition, activity, and profitability. The common ratios applicable to each of these areas will be discussed and current managerial issues illustrated via the case of Community Medical Center. For this purpose, the balance sheets and statements of revenue and expense for 1977 and 1978 for Community Medical Center are reproduced from Chapter 2 as Exhibits 8–1, 8–2, and 8–3.

The reader should understand that ratios are merely the result of dividing one numerical value on the balance sheet or statement of revenues and expenses by another value. It is the analysis and managerial use of these ratios that are important. Moreover, ratios and relationships other than those presented here may be more useful, depending on particular circumstances. Thus the reader should be concerned not only with the common ratios presented here but also with the expandability of the concept of ratio analysis.

TYPES OF RATIOS

Liquidity Ratios

Liquidity is a measure of the institution's ability to convert assets into specific amounts of cash. Cash is the most liquid asset. Capital assets are relatively illiquid. Between these extremes are assets with various levels of liquidity. By major balance sheet category, current assets are the most liquid of assets. However, a true measure of an institution's liquidity can be made only by comparing current assets to current amounts owed, current liabilities. Thus, the primary measure of a hospital's liquidity is the current ratio:

$$\frac{\text{Current assets (CA)}}{\text{Current liabilities (CL)}}$$

Because liquidity is an important factor in measuring a hospital's ability to cover current liabilities, questions arise as to the varying degrees of liquidity in the current asset section of the balance sheet. Obviously, cash is liquid, and receivables are current sources of cash. However, inventories and prepaid expenses are not necessarily as liquid on a cash conversion basis. Therefore, a more strict measure of liquidity has developed—the acid test ratio:

$$\frac{\text{Cash + Net accounts receivable (C+NAR)}}{\text{Current liabilities (CL)}}$$

The ultimate measure of liquidity is cash. Cash includes cash, checking, savings accounts, and "liquid" investments such as treasury bills. Thus, the ultimate measure of liquidity as previously defined in a ratio format is:

$$\frac{\text{Cash (C)}}{\text{Current liabilities (CL)}}$$

Exhibit 8-1 Community Medical Center: Balance Sheet Assets, for the Years 1977 and 1978 Ending December 31

	1978	1977
	(in 000s)	
Current Assets:		
Cash	$ 13	$ 100
Receivables, less reserves for uncollectable accounts and contractual allowances of $995,000 and $885,000	2,941	2,508
Inventories	297	332
Prepaid insurance	31	15
Total current assets	$ 3,282	$ 2,955
Property, Plant, and Equipment, at cost:		
Land	$ 579	$ 503
Land improvements	285	265
Buildings and building service equipment	16,604	16,545
Departmental equipment	2,979	2,771
Construction in progress	553	28
	$21,000	$20,112
Less accumulated depreciation	7,057	5,938
	$13,943	$14,174
Other Assets:		
Unamortized debt expense	$ 79	$ 96
Board-designated funds for plant expansion:		
Treasury bills	1,632	1,430
	$ 1,711	$ 1,526
	$18,936	$18,655
Restricted Funds		
Industrial Development Fund:		
Due from unrestricted fund	$ 20	$ —
	$ 20	$ —

Exhibit 8-2 Community Medical Center: Balance Sheet Liabilities and Fund Balances, for the Years 1977 and 1978 Ending December 31

	1978	1977
	(in 000s)	
Current Liabilities:		
Current maturities of long-term debt	$ 320	$ 295
Note payable, 12%	10	15
Accounts payable	910	524
Accrued liabilities	595	595
Other reserves	24	18
Due to restricted fund	20	—
Total current liabilities	$ 1,879	$ 1,447
Deferred Revenues, arising from use of accelerated depreciation for Medicare and Medicaid reimbursement	$ 356	$ 340
Long-Term Debt, less current maturities	$ 5,500	$ 6,000
Fund Balance	$11,201	$10,868
	$18,936	$18,655
Restricted Funds		
Industrial Development Fund:		
Fund balance	$ 20	$ —
	$ 20	$ —

Exhibit 8–3 Community Medical Center: Statements of Revenues and Expenses, for the Years 1977 and 1978 Ending December 31

	1978	1977
	(in 000s)	
Operating Revenue:		
Gross revenue from patient services:		
Inpatient	$14,513	$12,468
Outpatient	1,458	1,303
	$15,971	$13,771
Revenue deductions	1,510	1,599
Net revenue from patient services	$14,461	$12,172
Other operating revenue	222	179
Total operating revenue	$14,683	$12,351
Operating Expenses:		
Salaries	$ 7,045	$ 5,773
Fees and commissions	1,379	1,193
Supplies	2,748	2,103
Other expenses	1,753	1,178
Interest and amortization of debt expense	520	549
Depreciation-cost	1,125	1,139
Total operating expenses	$14,570	$11,935
Income (loss) from operations	$ 113	$ 416
Nonoperating Revenue:		
Contributions	21	9
Interest income	143	149
Excess (deficiency) of revenues over expenses	$ 277	$ 574

As an analysis tool, the higher the liquidity ratio, the more liquid the institution's financial position. It is the responsibility of the hospital's administration to establish basic guidelines for absolute or relative movement towards specified liquidity goals. As much cash as possible should be invested in revenue-producing operations—including investments. Also, a consistent decision must be made as to the classification of funded depreciation. A case may be made that such restricted funds are not readily available for current operations and therefore should be excluded from liquidity ratio computations. However, if board-restricted, such funds are under the control of the hospital, and, as a practical matter, liabilities would be paid from these funds if no other recourse were available. Thus, a case could be made that funds such as funded depreciation should be included in liquidity measurements.

In reference to Community Medical Center, we find current assets equal to $3,281,863 for 1978 and current liabilities equal to $1,878,292. Therefore, the current ratio is 1.747 ($3,281,863 ÷ $1,878,292). If funded depreciation were added to current assets, current assets would equal $5,086,863 ($3,281,863 + $1,805,000), with a corresponding current ratio of 2.708. Whether or not funded depreciation is added to current assets depends on the particular circumstances of the institution. However, inclusion or exclusion of these funds must be consistent between comparison periods to evaluate liquidity movements adequately. For present purposes, funded depreciation will not be added to current assets.

Thus, the acid test ratio for Community Medical Center for 1978 is computed as follows:

$$\text{Acid test ratio} = \frac{CC + NAR}{CL} = \frac{\$13,034 + \$2,941,040}{\$1,878,292} = 1.57$$

The absolute liquidity ratio of C/CL is 0.00694 ($13,034/$1,878,292). At this point, the reader should compute the liquidity ratios of Community Medical Center for 1977 and compare them to those of 1978.

Leverage Ratios

Leverage has as its basis the use of borrowed funds in financing assets. It is possible to acquire, via the incurrence of debt, assets in excess of internally generated funds as reflected in the fund balance. Generally, debt is serviced over an extended period of time, resulting in expanded current operations with debt servicing from future operations. Leverage is a powerful tool in the expansion of operations and the financing of assets. However, the overextension of the hospital could lead to severe liquidity problems and possible bankruptcy if the debt cannot be serviced from future operations.

Leverage relates to the amount of assets that are financed by operations as reflected in the fund balance. One common measure of leverage is the ratio:

$$\frac{\text{Total assets (TA)}}{\text{Fund balance (FB)}}$$

Leverage may also be visualized as the use of long-term debt rather than operating reserves in financing assets. Thus, a second leverage ratio may be developed:

$$\frac{\text{Long-term debt (LTD)}}{\text{Fund balance (FB)}}$$

A third leverage measure, related to the above ratios, is the relationship of total assets to long-term debt: $\text{TA} = \text{TA} \times \text{LTD}$, which ties the three liquidity measures together.

From a managerial perspective, the risk of incurring extensive debt must be weighed against the advantages of increased operational capacity, fixed amounts of debt service for extended periods of time, and the use of external funds in financing current operations. Relative to 1978 leverage for Community Medical Center, the computations of the three leverage ratios are as follows:

$$\frac{\text{TA}}{\text{FB}} = \frac{\$19,108,661}{\$11,664,675} = 1.63$$

$$\frac{\text{LTD}}{\text{FB}} = \frac{\$5,209,915}{\$11,664,675} = 0.447$$

$$\frac{\text{TA}}{\text{FB}} = \frac{\text{TA}}{\text{LTD}} \times \frac{\text{LTD}}{\text{FB}}$$

Therefore, $\dfrac{\text{TA}}{\text{LTD}} = \dfrac{\text{TA}}{\text{FB}} \times \dfrac{1}{(\text{LTD/FB})} = 1.63 \times 1/0.447 = 3.65.$

From a long-range viewpoint, if programs are developed that meet cost/benefit criteria, there is the potential for increased use of leverage via debt. In the case of the center, there is also the possibility of a major construction program. Assuming an incurrence of $20 million in long-term debt, the impact on the financials and leverage ratios would be as follows:

Total Assets = $19,108,661 + $20,000,000 = $39,108,661,
Long-Term Debt = $5,209,915 + $20,000,000 = $25,209,915,

therefore,

$$\frac{\text{TA}}{\text{FB}} = \frac{\$39,108,661}{\$11,664,675} = 3.35,$$

$$\frac{\text{LTD}}{\text{FB}} = \frac{\$25,209,915}{\$11,664,675} = 2.16,$$

and

$$\frac{TA}{FB} = 3.35 \times (1/2.16) = 1.55,$$

or

$$\frac{LTD}{TA} = 1/1.55 = 0.644.$$

Note the alterations in the ratios relative to leverage utilization. Obviously, a substantially greater proportion of assets is financed by the incurrence of debt. The issue of whether or not this is a sounder financial position depends in large part on the "soundness" of current and projected operations that are not evidenced by the leverage ratios alone.

Composition Ratios

As noted above, varying degrees of liquidity and variations are possible by segregating terms to determine the effects on the ability of the institution to cover its current liabilities. Extending our analysis to the entire list of asset categories, it is managerially important to determine the composition of assets. For this purpose, a series of useful common ratios have been developed.

For the three major asset sections in the balance sheet—current, fixed, and other—the initial composition ratios are:

$$\frac{\text{Current assets (CA)}}{\text{Total assets (TA)}}$$

$$\frac{\text{Fixed assets (FA)}}{\text{Total assets (TA)}}$$

$$\frac{\text{Other assets (OA)}}{\text{Total assets (TA)}}$$

The sum of these ratios is equal to one; therefore, the analyst is able to identify the split of assets into the major sections. This split is managerially useful because it permits the identification of major shifts of asset composition over time. If a major construction program is anticipated at some point in the future, the goals of the institution should be to increase funds available for the program. Thus, both liquidity and flexibility should be emphasized in financial planning, with some assets moving toward current and other asset accounts rather than toward fixed asset accounts.

Similarly, it is informative to identify components of current assets. As noted, current asset components have varying degrees of liquidity, with cash being the most liquid. From this fact, a second series of composition ratios have been developed:

$$\frac{\text{Other current assets (OCA)}}{\text{Total current assets (TCA)}}$$

$$\frac{\text{Inventory (INV)}}{\text{Total current assets (TCA)}}$$

$$\frac{\text{Total accounts receivable (TAR)}}{\text{Total current assets (TCA)}}$$

$$\frac{\text{Cash (C)}}{\text{Total current assets (TCA)}}$$

The analyst must be in a position to evaluate the composition of current assets in line with the financial requirements of the institution relative to liquidity. A growing trend in receivables, inventory, and other current assets is to require evaluation of the underlying circumstances of these increases. A high proportion of current assets in noncash items greatly reduces the flexibility and potential of the institution to expand operations and cover current liabilities.

Similarly, at least a simple analysis must be made of receivables relative to total receivables and net receivables. A clearer picture of receivables management is provided by reducing total receivables by reserves for contractual allowances, uncollectable accounts, and amounts that are not directly related to patient accounts receivables performance under the control of the hospital's business office, such as receivables due from cost reporting, physicians' rentals, and so on.

From the balance sheet of Community Medical Center, the following composition ratios may be computed for 1978:

$$\frac{\text{Current assets}}{\text{Total assets}} = \frac{\$3,281,863}{\$19,108,661} = 0.1717$$

$$\frac{\text{Fixed assets}}{\text{Total assets}} = \frac{\$13,943,178}{\$19,108,661} = 0.7297$$

$$\frac{\text{Other assets}}{\text{Total assets}} = \frac{\$1,883,620}{\$19,108,661} = 0.0986$$

Note that the sum $0.1717 + 0.7297 + 0.0986 = 1.0000$.

For the composition of current assets, the following ratios are derived:

$$\frac{\text{Other current assets}}{\text{Total current assets}} = \frac{\$31,048}{\$3,281,863} = 0.0095$$

$$\frac{\text{Inventory}}{\text{Total current assets}} = \frac{\$296,741}{\$3,281,863} = 0.0904$$

$$\frac{\text{Total accounts receivable}}{\text{Total current assets}} = \frac{\$2,941,040 + \$995,300}{\$3,281,863} = 1.199$$

$$\frac{\text{Net accounts receivable}}{\text{Total accounts receivable}} = \frac{\$2,941,040}{\$2,941,040 + \$995,300} = 0.7472$$

$$\frac{\text{Cash}}{\text{Total current assets}} = \frac{\$13,034}{\$3,281,863} = 0.0040$$

For purposes of analysis, these ratios must be evaluated in terms of planning criteria and prior-period levels. However, a general evaluation reveals a high level of asset mix in fixed assets and a relatively illiquid current asset position, given the large receivable component. Note that the gross receivables resulting from reserves and net receivables are almost equal to the entire amount of current assets. (Note: In the above computation, an allowance was not made for extraordinary receivables in the calculation of net receivables, due to the payable position of the medical center for Medicare, Medicaid, and Blue Cross.) In order to enhance its current position, the center would be required to utilize debt or to "borrow" internally from funded depreciation.

From this analysis, it appears that future managerial action should be related to the enhancement of receivables management with a goal of strengthening the liquidity position of the institution. The potential for incurring significant amounts of debt is risky in the short term. If bonds are expected to be floated in 1980 for the expansion program, a critical year of operations is 1979. Enhancements in the liquidity of the center will strengthen the appearance of sound fiscal management, even though cash flow cannot improve to a significant extent. An indication of sound managerial action and guidance would be to go into the 1980 construction program with a comfortable amount of internally generated funds.

This underscores again the need for hospitals to be guided by long-range financial and operational planning. Such planning by Community Medical Center would lead to a liquidity management program with enhanced levels of funds available for expansion.

Activity Ratios

To this point, we have been concerned with the positional aspects of a hospital's financial operations. However, it is essential to interface operating results with financial position to identify relationships indicating the effects of current operations on the institution's financial position. The common ratio series relative to operations rather than with position are called activity ratios, a subset of which is turnover ratios. Turnover ratios are generally related to revenue and balance sheet items. For example, inventory turnover is defined as operating revenue divided by average inventory, which provides an indication of how many times during the period the total inventory was used in operations. Activity ratios compare operations over a period of time with items reported at the end of the period. Consequently, a more reasonable comparison is possible when average balances are used for balance sheet items in computing the activity ratio. A simple average of (beginning balance + ending balance)/2 is a useful approximation of the average amount of the balance sheet item. The following are commonly used activity ratios:

$$\text{Asset turnover} = \frac{\text{Operating revenue (OR)}}{\text{Average total assets (ATA)}}$$

$$\text{Miscellaneous asset turnover} = \frac{\text{Operating revenue (OR)}}{\text{Average miscellaneous assets (AMA)}}$$

$$\text{Fixed asset turnover} = \frac{\text{Operating revenue (OR)}}{\text{Average fixed assets (AFA)}}$$

$$\text{Current asset turnover} = \frac{\text{Operating revenue (OR)}}{\text{Average current assets (ACA)}}$$

$$\text{Inventory turnover} = \frac{\text{Operating revenue (OR)}}{\text{Average inventory (AI)}}$$

$$\text{Total receivables turnover} = \frac{\text{Operating revenue (OR)}}{\text{Average total receivables (ATR)}}$$

$$\text{Days in accounts receivable} = \frac{\text{Average total accounts receivables}}{\text{(Operating revenue/Days in period)}}$$

$$= \text{Days in period/Total receivables turnover}$$

$$\text{Days in net accounts receivables} = \text{Days in period/Net receivables turnover}$$

$$= \frac{\text{Average net accounts receivables}}{\text{(Operating revenue (OR)/Days in period)}}$$

$$\text{Net receivables turnover} = \frac{\text{Operating revenue (OR)}}{\text{Average net accounts receivables}}$$

$$\text{Cash turnover} = \frac{\text{Operating revenue (OR)}}{\text{Cash (C)}}$$

From an analytical viewpoint, the turnover ratios relate to the efficiency in utilizing assets in operations of the institution. The asset turnover ratio is a measure of the assets utilized in the hospital's operations. The higher the revenue generated per asset unit, the more effectively the assets are being utilized.

Of particular interest in the hospital field are the ratios related to receivables. Historically, days in accounts receivable has been a key measure of the operational efficiency of a hospital's patient accounting system. Further refinements of the receivables ratios may be developed by class of payer and patient demographics.

The following are computations of activity ratios for 1978 operations of Community Medical Center:

$$\text{Asset turnover} = \frac{\text{Operating revenue}}{(\text{Beginning assets} + \text{Ending assets})/2}$$

$$= \frac{\$14,683,127}{(\$18,654,934 + \$19,108,661)/2} = 0.7776$$

$$\text{Miscellaneous asset turnover} = \frac{\$14,683,127}{(\$1,526,269 + \$1,883,620)/2} = 8.6121$$

$$\text{Fixed asset turnover} = \frac{\$14,683,127}{(\$13,943,178 + \$14,174,025)/2} = 1.0444$$

$$\text{Current asset turnover} = \frac{\$14,683,127}{(\$3,281,863 + \$2,954,640)/2} = 4.7087$$

$$\text{Inventory turnover} = \frac{\$14,683,127}{(\$296,741 + \$331,813)/2} = 46.72$$

$$\text{Total receivables turnover} = \frac{\$14,683,127}{(\$2,941,040 + \$995,300 + \$2,507,722 + \$885,300)/2}$$
$$= 4.0066$$

$$\text{Days in accounts receivable} = \frac{\text{Days in period}}{\text{Total receivables turnover}} = 365/4.0066 = 91.1000$$

$$\text{Net receivables turnover} = \frac{\$14,683,127}{(\$2,941,040 + \$2,507,722)/2} = 5.3895$$

$$\text{Days in net accounts receivables} = \frac{\text{Days in period}}{\text{Net receivables turnover}} = \frac{365}{5.3895} = 67.72$$

Other activity ratios may be developed to relate current liabilities to operating items such as operating expenses net of depreciation. Such relationships are useful for planning purposes and the identification of trends in the utilization of debt in financing operations.

Profitability Ratios

It is not only important to identify relationships that indicate financial position and asset utilization, it is also essential to identify ratios that show what returns are earned on investment and how profitable operations are. With profitability measures as a basis, the following ratios have been developed for general use:

$$\text{Return on fund balance} = \frac{\text{Net income (NI)}}{\text{Beginning fund balance (BFB)}}$$

$$\text{Return on total assets} = \frac{\text{Net income (NI)}}{\text{Total assets (TA)}}$$

$$\text{Net profit margin} = \frac{\text{Net income (NI)}}{\text{Operating revenue (OR)}}$$

$$\text{Net versus operating income} = \frac{\text{Net income (NI)}}{\text{Operating income (OI)}}$$

$$\text{Operating return on total assets} = \frac{\text{Operating income (OI)}}{\text{Beginning total assets (BTA)}}$$

$$\text{Debt coverage} = \frac{\text{Net income + Depreciation + Interest expense}}{\text{Debt service}}$$

These ratios are intuitively appealing as measures of the profitability of operations. Returns on fund balance and total assets are measures of how effectively accumulated funds and assets are utilized in earning a profit for future asset replacements and enhancements. The net profit margin is a useful measure of operational relationships in the statement of revenues and expenses. The operating ratio of operating expenses + operating income is a possible expansion of the net profit margin. The operating ratio computed on a departmental basis is useful in identifying departmental profitability and adherence to budgeted levels.

Due to the nonoperating segments of hospital operations such as interest income, it is important to evaluate the profitability of operations alone. Therefore, two additional ratios—net versus operating income and operating return on total assets—have been developed as measures of the proportion of net income related solely to operations and to the effective use of assets in operations. Finally, a key operational and profitability measure used extensively in evaluating debt service capability is the debt coverage ratio, which relates to the ability of the hospital to service debt from operations. To provide a true measure of debt service capability, depreciation and interest are eliminated to approximate cash flow and to eliminate the effects of current interest expense. Thus, the amount of cash flow before debt is compared to total annual debt service. A debt coverage ratio of 1.5 to 1.0 is considered a reasonable level of coverage, though circumstances will dictate the required figure.

The profitability ratios for 1978 for Community Medical Center are computed as follows:

$$\text{Return on fund balance} = \frac{(\$54,008)}{\$11,331,801} = (0.0477)$$

$$\text{Return on total assets} = \frac{(\$54,008)}{\$18,654,934} = (0.0029)$$

$$\text{Net profit margin} = \frac{(\$54,008)}{\$14,683,127} = (0.0037)$$

$$\text{Net versus operating income} = \frac{(\$54,008)}{(\$218,722)} = 0.2469$$

$$\text{Operating return on total assets} = \frac{(\$218,722)}{\$18,654,934} = (0.01172)$$

$$\text{Debt coverage ratio} = \frac{(\$54,008) + \$520,208 + \$1,124,877 + \$330,856}{\$295,000 + \$520,208} = 2.3576$$

(Note: $295,000 is the current maturity of long-term debt.)

An analysis of the above ratios indicates a negative profitability from overall operations and a significant loss from patient operations. However, price level depreciation has a significant impact on operating results, and debt coverage is relatively strong from a modified cash flow standpoint. While these ratios must be compared with historic activities and planned levels, it appears that Community Medical Center has the ability to service increased debt. However, it appears that net income for future inflation has not been adequately generated in light of the relatively aggressive expansion program.

INDUSTRY DATA AND UTILIZATION OF RATIOS

Commercial industries have historically utilized ratios as bases in developing industry-wide averages to serve as norms for internal use. While industry averages must be analyzed and used in the light of a particular company's operating environment, such norms are also useful in basic financial analysis. The hospital industry has not developed industry-wide data formulated as hospital average ratios on a formal basis. The unique circumstances surrounding the many different operations of a particular hospital hinder normative ratio average generation. With patient care as the main "product" of the hospital, it is difficult to identify the average hospital. Each hospital and each patient is unique, involving an extremely wide range of services and needs within each operating environment.

Despite the current lack of valid industry data, however, ratio analysis is an effective analytical tool and structure around which financial evaluation and planning can be built. The hospital analyst should develop trend comparisons of ratios over a number of years and relate these trends to an overall, long-range financial planning and evaluation system governed by the goals and objectives of the organization. The development of such a comprehensive financial model requires an indepth understanding of the components of hospital finance and the basic objectives and operations of the institution on both an historic and forecasted basis.

COMMUNITY MEDICAL CENTER: APPLICATION OF RATIO ANALYSIS

The reader at this point should begin to formalize financial relationships for Community Medical Center for historic operations. Also, the reader should begin to organize and associate data in at least a subjective analysis of the overall direction that the center should take in the future with regard to expansion plans and the need for strong managerial action to achieve some of the institution's basic objectives.

The reader, again in the role of president of Community Medical Center, should develop ratios and comparisons for the years 1977 to 1979 from the financial data presented in Chapters 5, 6, and 7. From these trend data, an action plan should be developed focused on the following:

- What areas of Community Medical Center's operations require managerial intervention?

- In these areas, what should be the general direction of the action taken?

- From the above analysis, develop an overall organizational strategy that relates managerial financial actions to the proposed expansion program.

Chapter 9

Working Capital Management

INTRODUCTION

In today's operating environment, the hospital must be extremely concerned with its liquidity position and its ability effectively to manage components of its current assets and related current liabilities. In previous discussion we identified working capital as current assets minus current liabilities and developed several ratios to identify relationships of current assets and components to total assets and operating results. At this point, it is appropriate to identify key managerial issues related to the working capital components of receivables, inventory, payables, cash, and insurance.

Our discussion begins with a managerial analysis of receivables, including the essential aspects of effective receivables administration. Receivables are the largest segment of the general hospital's current assets. Generally, almost all of a hospital's revenue generation is in the form of credit at the time of service. Consequently, the speed, accuracy, and efficiency with which receivables are turned into cash directly affect the liquidity position of the institution.

While inventories are a relatively small proportion of a hospital's assets, it is possible to identify managerial techniques for the effective management of inventories. Having already examined last-in-first-out (LIFO) and first-in-first-out (FIFO) procedures and periodic and perpetual accounting practices, our examination of inventories in the present chapter will identify economic order quantities and safety stock and will illustrate specific quantitative techniques in their application to financial systems.

Payables as a liability are a method of financing assets. Normal accounts payable are amounts of short-term financing related to the acquisition of goods or services. It is important to analyze purchase agreements for the terms of payment. Often terms such as 2/10, net 30 are used. In this example, the terms provide for a 2 percent discount if payment is made within 10 days after billing, and full payment is due within 30 days at a loss of the discount. Usually, finance charges are made for late payment. Our concern in the present chapter is with the costs and benefits associated with the timing of payables payments and with the key managerial elements of this mode of financing assets.

In our discussion of cash, we will examine the various investment vehicles that are available for short-term investment, such as treasury bills, certificates of deposit, and repurchase agreements.

Finally, insurance principles and practices in the context of working capital management will be discussed. Insurance coverage is essential for the protection of all assets and operations of the institution. It is important that the hospital administration understand the basic concepts and operations of property insurance, malpractice insurance, and other insurance coverages. In this section, coinsurance terms and key managerial issues will be identified.

KEY COMPONENTS

Receivables

The management of receivables must be directly supervised at the highest levels of the institution via goals, policies, and procedures established as a part of the revenue cycle. The responsibility for implementing credit policies and operating procedures related to receivables generally rests with the business office.

Effective receivables management is the result of strict adherence to the basic credit philosophy that cash flow is directly related to the speed and accuracy of the initial billing information and to the communications associated with credit follow-up. Figure 9–1 illustrates the basic steps in the flow of patient information through the business office functions of admitting, data collection, billing, and credit/collection. While the diagram is oversimplified, the key areas for managerial interfacing with policies and procedures can be identified.

Admitting

The first areas in which a patient comes into direct contact with the hospital are admitting, outpatient/clinic, and emergency room. At these points the direct collection activities should begin. Even before a patient comes to the hospital, collection information may be gathered through an advance registration or preadmission process. The steps for preadmission are:

- The admitting physician contacts the admitting area, stating that a particular patient is to be admitted on or around a specific date and/or time.

- The admitting area schedules the patient by reserving a bed for the admission date.

- The admitting area contacts the patient by phone and/or mail, requesting basic admitting information regarding insurance coverage, demographic date, and so forth.

- Insurance coverage is verified by someone in the business office.

- Additional contacts may then be made with the patient, describing coverage and setting up payment arrangements even prior to admission.

Data Collection

An effective preadmission program requires continuous communication and cooperation in the exchange of data with the physician and the physician's office. Many times the condition of the patient precludes preadmission. At the time of the patient's initial contact with the hospital, it is imperative that complete and accurate information be obtained and that the institution's credit policies be explained to the patient or the patient's representative. Consequently, it is essential that personnel in the emergency room, outpatient/clinic, and admitting areas be familiar with insurance coverage and data requirements so that full information is obtained before service is rendered.

For inpatient stays, patient data should flow to the persons responsible for billing and patient follow-up. Third party coverage should be verified, and the completeness and accuracy of the data should be checked while the patient is in-house. Either while the patient is in-house or at time of discharge, any missing data should be obtained, necessary arrangements should be made regarding the self-pay portion of the bill. All self-pay amounts should be referred to the credit/collection area for the setting up of payment arrangements.

Outpatient services, though representing only a small proportion of the average hospital's revenue, produce a significant data flow through the business office. Historically, if payment or valid insurance is not obtained at the time of service, it has been difficult to collect from the patient after the service is rendered. An increasing number of hospitals are therefore investigating the method of requiring payment from the patient and not billing third parties for outpatient services. Such an alteration in practice requires managerial decision making in the areas of public relations, costs of billing, and potential impacts on cash flow.

Figure 9-1 Business Office Data Flow

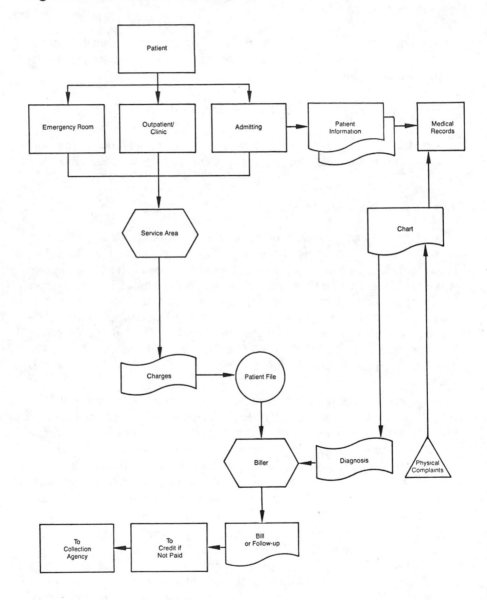

Billing, Credit, and Collection

One of the most difficult areas to manage effectively is the credit department, including relationships with outside agencies such as banks and collection agencies. At the time an account is determined to be a self-pay, the credit department should become actively involved in the collection of the account. Arrangements should be made between the hospital and the patient for a mutually agreeable payment schedule. If the terms of potential patient payment are projected over a significant period of time, many hospitals utilize bank notes, which results in the hospital receiving payment while the patient and bank develop a payment schedule. Care should be taken in dealing with such bank notes to ensure that the note is without recourse to the hospital. This means that the patient is fully responsible for payment to the bank and that, if default occurs, the hospital is not liable to the bank for any portion of the unpaid balance.

Another relationship that has developed between banks and hospitals involves factoring accounts. In factoring receivables, the hospital "sells" accounts to an external agency such as a bank at a discount. The patient then pays the bank with interest. The disadvantage of factoring lies in the usual practice of recourse in the factoring agreement. If the patient defaults on the account and the hospital has to "buy" the account back from the factoring agent, the hospital could lose the discount. A contingent liability must be established on the financial statements for accounts that may have to be "bought" back by the hospital.

Finally, the use of outside collection agencies has become an attractive means for hospitals to deal with accounts that are uncollectable by the internal system. At the time the account is turned over to the collection agency, it is recorded as a bad debt by the hospital. As collections are made by the agency, the amounts collected are recorded as recoveries of bad debts in total, and the collection fee is recorded as a current operating expense. In selecting a collection agency, the hospital must be concerned not only with the collection fee but also with the effectiveness and basic operating ethics and policies of the agency in line with hospital philosophy. Collection agencies are useful collection tools for hospitals because they can fully investigate an account, follow up in accordance with fair credit legislation, and sue or garnish wages as an "independent" party separate from the hospital. However, the hospital's consent for each account action is required.

In selecting and dealing with a collection agency, the hospital must first decide on the number of agencies to utilize. Often the competitive environment created through the use of two or more agencies produces more effective collection operations. The relationships and communications between the collection agency and the hospital must be on an open and efficient basis. Past hospital experience and rates are important factors in dealing with the agency. References should be explored. A periodic bid basis for selecting agencies requires effective relationships between the hospital and the agencies as to rates and operating practices.

The data flow from nonpatient areas must be accurate and timely. Patient charges should be posted on a daily basis that eliminates billing cut-off problems, such as late charges or period-end errors in revenue reporting. Data from medical records are often required before a bill can be sent. Such data include discharge diagnoses and the coding of diagnosis and treatment procedures in line with the ICD–9 international coding of diseases. In practice, the accumulation of these data depends on completed charts and direct physician involvement in patient charting. Often, charts are not completed on a basis that is timely enough for billing. In such cases, it is imperative that each bit of insurance data be analyzed and that alternative means be developed for a more rapid flow of data into the billing system. It may even be necessary to make a person from the business office responsible for the billing data flow from such supporting areas as medical records.

Patient Representatives

The data flows we have described relate to a traditional business office organizational structure. However, the actual organization of the business office will vary, depending to a large extent on the environmental circumstances. An increasing number of hospitals have moved to a patient representative organization. The full patient representative system provides that a single person handle all patient data and contacts from admission to final payment or write-off. Generally, the work is divided among office personnel, based on division of patients' names by alphabet. The advantages of this system are:

- Consistent patient contact and full centralization of patient data are possible.

- With such centralization, problem areas can be quickly identified and corrective action taken.

- The patients have a single contact person who is familiar with all aspects of the patients' individual situations and with whom they can correspond.

There are, however, also disadvantages of the patient representative system:

- Each patient representative must be familiar with several insurance companies and related billing procedures.

- Managerial control of specific segments of data flowing through the office is more difficult.

- If a representative quits or is ill, it is often difficult to replace the personal expertise represented by existing patient files.

Modifications of the patient representative system have been successfully adapted to the hospital's specific operating environment. In some cases, patient representatives are utilized only in billing commercial insurance, with admitting, credit, and special accounts (Medicare and Medicaid) established as traditional structures. Here, the patient representatives are used for the billing and follow-up on those patients with commercial insurance. Whatever method is used, the policies and procedures must be formulated with speed, accuracy, and communication as the basic objectives.

Management Reporting

With respect to management reporting, it is essential that administrative personnel and those responsible for the management of the business office identify and monitor the following key elements of business office operations that indicate levels of performance:

- gross receivable balances

- receivables activity, for example, charge collections by carrier, and bad debts by carrier and area, such as inpatient, outpatient, and emergency room

- days to bill by carrier and daily billing activity

- details of personnel activity

- physician statistics

Of course, just one overall figure, such as days in receivables, cannot represent the entire receivables management picture. Further detail is necessary so that full compliance with policies and procedures may be verified, potential problem areas identified, and corrective action taken.

Application to Community Medical Center

To illustrate the application of management reporting to business office operations, Tables 9–1 to 9–7 present forms used by the business office manager of Community Medical Center to evaluate the performance of the office's personnel. The manager reports to the controller's office daily cash flow and days in receivables.

Table 9-1 Community Medical Center: Billing and Collection Analysis

Party Billed	% of Total Billings	Days to Collect
Medicaid		
Medicare		
Other insurers		
Blue Cross		

Table 9-2 Community Medical Center: Evaluation of Collection Effort at Discharge for an Eight-Day Period

Total billings
  Third party billings
  Self-pay portion
    Collection at discharge
  Discharge collection effort
    Percent of total billings
    Percent of self-pay billings

Table 9-3 Community Medical Center: Income—Accounts Receivable

	1977	1978	% Increase
G/L accounts receivable balance			
G/L gross charges			
Patient days			

Table 9–4 Community Medical Center: Analysis for Billings and Collection Studies—30 Day Period

	Other Ins.	Self-Pay	Medicare	Medicaid
Number of billings				
Average/billing				
Average number of days from discharge to billing				
Average number of days from billing to payment				
Average number of days to collect self-pay portion				
Average amount of self-pay portion				

Table 9–5 Community Medical Center: Study of Self-Pay Collections for a 30-Day Period

Number of Accounts	1977 $ Value	%	1978 $ Value	%
Paid within 30 days				
Paid within 60 days				
Current contracts				
Bank notes				
Bad debts				
Totals				

Table 9–6 Community Medical Center: Comparison of Income with Collections

	1977	1978
Gross charges		
Cash collections		
Percentage of collections to income		

Table 9–7 Community Medical Center: Bad Debt Comparisons—
Emergency and Outpatient

	1977	1978
Total revenue		
Bad debts		
Percentage of bad debts to total revenue		

Based on the previous chapter's analysis of receivables, the reader should now be able to develop a comprehensive management reporting program for the evaluation of the center's business office operations. The initial task is the evaluation of the formats of Tables 9–1 to 9–7 in the light of the reader's perceived management information needs.

Inventory

Although the dollar amount of inventories constitutes a relatively small proportion of a hospital's total assets, it is an area where adequate controls and the application of related techniques can provide for some cost containment and for increased levels of cash flow control and managerial effectiveness. Historically, hospitals have accumulated significant amounts of medical supplies and drugs in areas like central supply, operating room, pharmacy, laboratory, and storeroom. Other areas, such as maintenance, housekeeping, laundry, and dietary, also accumulate supplies used in the supporting services of the hospital.

The basis for supply purchases is usually found in orders of the medical staff or in an obvious need for the desired items. Pressures for supplies needed to run the institution often result in the acquisition and storage of significant amounts of material with little thought given to the economics of the transactions. Optimally, the institution should determine systematically the need for the supplies and the quantities to order and should ensure that stockouts will not occur.

Certain managerial and quantitative techniques can lead to an increased degree of inventory control. These include purchasing and inventory systems procedures, the computation of economic order quantities, and safety stock level determination.

First, materials management systems must be developed to ensure operational efficiency in the acquisition and storage of supplies. As previously noted, the higher the degree of centralization of purchasing and storage operations, the greater the efficiency and control. An effective materials management system includes the following elements:

- The ordering of supplies should be centralized in as few areas as possible.

- The storage of supplies should be centralized in specific areas of the hospital where the supplies are dispensed.

- Perpetual inventory procedures should be utilized whenever possible, with allowance for a physical inventory at least once each year.

- Computations of economic order quantities and safety stock should be made for large-volume, high-cost items.

In short, the key elements of a materials management system involve the positioning of supply acquisition and storage in a centralized location in the hospital where quantitative techniques may be applied to the identification of economic order quantities and safety stock levels. Supplies of course incur costs in storage and ordering. The larger the quantity of supplies ordered, the less frequently they must be ordered. Hence, acquisition costs are reduced as the quantity ordered becomes larger. However, the larger the quantity of goods ordered, the higher the storage costs incurred. The computation of the economic order quantity identifies the optimum quantity of goods to order, given the quantity used in a specified period of time. The following example illustrates the computation of the economic order quantity (EOQ).

Assume that a quantity Q of supplies is used in a period of time T and that the usage is uniform over the period. Figure 9–2 illustrates the uniform usage pattern.

Given this pattern, the average quantity stored is Q/2. If the storage cost C_s is developed on a per unit basis, the average storage costs for the period are $C_s \times (Q_o/2)$, where Q_o is the quantity ordered. If the acquisition costs are identified as C_p, we have the total acquisition cost of $C_p \times (Q/Q_o)$, where Q is the usage of the supply and Q_o is the quantity ordered. Therefore, Q/Q_o is the number of times goods are ordered in the period.

The total inventory cost T_c is then $(C_s \times Q_o/2) + (C_p \times Q/Q_o)$. By determining the lowest point on the cost curve, one may determine the optimum Q_o for the least cost. From calculus, we know that the first derivative of T_c relative to Q_o provides the minimum point on the cost curve defined by the T_c equation when the first derivative is set equal to zero.

From this, we have the following: $O = T^1_c/Q^1_o = C_s/2 - (C_pQ)/Q_o^2$. Therefore, $C_s/2 = (C_pQ)/Q_o^2$, $Q_o^2 = (2C_pQ)/C_s$, and $Q_o = EOQ = \sqrt{(2C_pQ)/C_s}$.

Figure 9-2 Uniform Inventory Usage

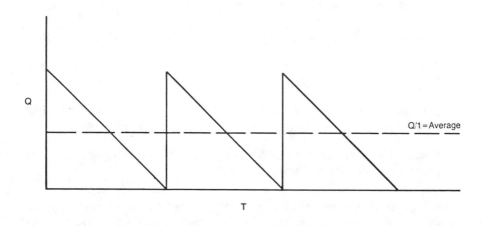

The case of Community Medical Center may be used to illustrate the EOQ computation. Assume that the center's laboratory used 5,000 cases of a reagent during 1978. To identify the necessary elements, one must compute C_p and C_s. The cost of purchasing these supplies includes a \$40,737 direct cost and a \$49,790 full cost. Storage costs include depreciation at \$5.28 per square foot, maintenance at \$1.37 per square foot, and operation of plant at \$2.38 per square foot. (Note that these costs may be criticized as being derived from the Medicare cost report based on adjusted costs. In the present case, their use can be justified in that they represent approximate measures of full cost and are easy to gather in the absence of more accurate full-cost data.) Assuming that Community Medical Center handled 10,000 orders in 1978 and that one case of reagent contains one cubic foot, we have the following costs and data elements: $Q = 5,000$; $C_p = \$40,737/10,000 = \$4.07$; $C_s = \$5.28 + \$1.37 + \$2.38 = \$9.03$. Inserting these data into the EOQ formula, we have: $EOQ = \sqrt{(2C_pQ)/C_s} = \sqrt{2(4.07)(5,000)/9.03} = \sqrt{4,507.20} = 67.13 \cong 68$ cases. Thus, the most economic size of an order is about 68 cases.

As a practical matter, stock should never be allowed to be completely depleted before an order is made, because of the lead time required to obtain new supplies. To prevent this, an appropriate level of safety stock should be determined. Safety stock is the minimum level of stock allowable before an order is placed. The ideal safety stock level depends on the following factors:

• the variability of expected inventory usage

- the length of time it takes to receive goods from the time they are ordered
- the size of the EOQ
- the criticality of the item in terms of patient care or facility operations.

These factors should be evaluated for historic trends and future projections. Assume that, in the case of Community Medical Center, the reagent usage in the laboratory is 5,000 units per year or 14 units per day. If it takes three days to receive a shipment, the safety stock level would be 3 × 14 or 42 units. If the safety stock level exceeds the EOQ, the safety stock level should serve as an adjustment to the EOQ. Usage variances must be taken into account when the safety stock level is computed.

The reader should at this point be able to run through the following data in computing the EOQ and safety stock for x-ray film at Community Medical Center. Assume that 10,000 cases of film are used, that a lead time of four days is required to receive film after an order is placed, and that one case of film takes two square feet of storage space.

Computerization must be considered for the calculation of EOQ and safety stock when there is a large number of items in a hospital's inventory. It is not uncommon for the pharmacy to have over 5,000 items in its inventory. More advanced quantitative techniques are available for the computation of safety stock based on expected usage during the time from order to receipt of the goods.

Insurance

While insurance coverage is not reflected in the current asset section of the balance sheet except through prepaid premium reporting, it is imperative that the hospital's operations and assets be adequately protected by insurance. Insurance coverages available to a hospital include fire and property damage, automobile, malpractice, and specific coverages on boilers, computers, and builder's risk. Public liability, workmen's compensation coverages, and various bondings for theft and business interruption are also available. As levels of debt incurred in the hospital industry have increased, there has been increasing emphasis on insurance coverages.

The extent of a hospital's fire and property damage coverage must be analyzed on an ongoing basis. The special terms and usage commonly used in property coverage policies must be understood to determine effectively the proper levels of coverage and to ensure that both overinsurance and underinsurance are avoided. It is important that detailed and up-to-date property records, including appraisals of replacement costs, are maintained. The use of deductibles is an effective way to reduce annual premiums, and a workable facility-maintenance and inspection program often can reduce risk factors, and thus also premiums. Generally, an insurance company will pay the smallest of the following amounts: (1) face value of the policy, (2) amount of loss, (3) a contribution limitation with multiple coverage, or (4) a coinsurance limitation.

To illustrate these limitations, suppose that in 1978 a small fire occurred in the warehouse of Community Medical Center. Two insurance companies are used for coverage of the hospital:

Insurance Company	Policy Face Total	Policy Face Warehouse	Coinsurance
A	$15,000,000	$40,000	90%
B	$20,000,000	$60,000	75%

Assume that the warehouse was built in 1970 at a cost of $100,000 with an estimated salvage value of $30,000 and an estimated life of 20 years. Straight-line depreciation is utilized for book purposes. A current appraisal lists the warehouse at a replacement cost of $125,000 with 60 percent having been destroyed by the fire. Therefore, the economic loss as a result of the fire was $125,000 × 60 percent = $75,000.

The face values of $40,000 and $60,000 are the limits of policies A and B respectively. A second limit is $75,000, the amount of the loss. Under a contribution limitation, the insurance company will not be liable for a greater proportion of any loss than the proportion of its insurance to the total amount covered. In this case, Company A would be liable for $40,000/$100,000 = 40 percent of the $75,000 loss or $30,000; Company B's limitation would be equal to $60,000/$100,000 = 60 percent of $75,000 or $45,000. Thus, $30,000 and $45,000 are the lesser figures for insurance coverage of policies A and B respectively.

Many property insurance policies contain a coinsurance clause requiring that the insured maintain contributing insurance on the property equal to at least a certain percentage of the actual cash value of the property at the time of the loss. If such contributing insurance is not maintained, the insured is liable to the extent of the deficit. The general coinsurance limitation formula is:

$$\frac{\text{Policy face}}{\text{Insurance required}} \times \text{Loss} = \text{Coinsurance limitation}$$

In the above case, the respective coinsurance limitations may be calculated as:

Company A: $40,000/(90% × $125,000) × $75,000 = $26,667
Company B: $60,000/(75% × $125,000) × $75,000 = $48,000

If all four limitations are in effect for both policies, Company A would pay $26,667 and Company B would pay $48,000 for a total recovery of $74,667. Depreciation on the building is $6,000 per year for eight years or $48,000. The entry to record the loss is:

	Debit	Credit
Cash	$74,667	
Accumulated depreciation ($48,000 × 60%)	$28,800	
Gain/loss from fire		$43,467
Buildings ($100,000 × 60%)		$60,000

Note that the economic loss from the fire is $75,000 less the recovery of $74,667 for a net economic loss of $333, even though a gain was realized for book purposes. This example illustrates the necessity for hospital administrators to understand the specific terminology in their insurance policies and to update coverage in line with current replacement values to the extent of the indicated limitations.

As an exercise, the reader may assume that the replacement value of the entire Community Medical Center complex is $40,000,000. From this, the reader should evaluate the adequacy of the coverage indicated in the above case, assuming the four common limitations are in effect.

Payables and Short-Term Financing

Accounts payable are, as we have seen, a source of short-term financing. Often, some form of discount is available for payment within a specified time period. Payments after this period result in the loss of the discount, which is in effect a cost for the use of payables as a source of funds. Even in the absence of a discount, the overextension of payables could result in the loss of credit availability and the imposition of finance charges by the creditors.

In the case of discount loss, the cost of trade credit may be quantified as follows:

$$C_t = (d/(1 - d) \times (365/e);$$
where: d = % of discount, and
e = Days after discount period when payment is made.

As an example, assume the following: terms of 2/10, net 30. This means a two percent discount is available if payment is made within 10 days, with the full amount due 30 days after the invoice date. Therefore:

- If payment is made at 30 days, $C_t = .02/(1 - .02) \times 365/20 = 0.372$. Here the cost of credit is 37.2 percent for the delay in payment.

- If payment is made at 60 days, $C_t = .02/(1 - .02) \times 365/50 = 0.149$.

- If payment is made at 90 days, $C_t = .02/(1 - .02) \times 365/80 = 0.093$.

This analysis of the use of payables in financing assets indicates that the longer the delay in payment, the lower the cost associated with the loss of the discount. If C_t, the cost associated with the discount loss, is less than the current borrowing rate or opportunity costs of investing in operations, the discount should be refused. In any case, a policy and formal analysis should be made related to the acceptance of discounts and the time periods for making payments in light of the particular circumstances of the hospital's cash and liquidity position.

Cash Investment Management

Sound financial management practice dictates that cash not be held in noninterest bearing checking accounts but rather invested in instruments that provide interest. The ideal situation would allow for cash deposits to be immediately invested in a savings account and to be withdrawn on an as-needed disbursement basis, with the funds earning interest from the time of deposit to the time of withdrawal. Cash receipts should be deposited on a daily basis, and the daily bank balance should be analyzed by a responsible person in the organization. The administration of the hospital should set goals for the amounts of funds held in cash accounts based on objective criteria, such as payroll needs and discount policies related to payables or as a percentage of historic operating expenses.

As we shall see in the following chapter, Medicare regulations require that interest income be offset against operating interest expense for amounts not designated as funded depreciation. The average hospital expends significant amounts of cash for asset replacement. Therefore, consideration should be given to funding depreciation in interest-bearing instruments to the highest amount possible. The maximum allowable by Medicare is the amount of accumulated depreciation.

Common instruments used for short-term investment include certificates of deposit (CDs), treasury bills, repurchase agreements, and savings accounts. Certificates of deposit are issued by banks for a specific period of time, usually a minimum of 30 days for a specified amount of interest. Interest rates vary somewhat from bank to bank and by amounts invested. The interest rates on CDs are generally higher than for other short-term instruments. On the other hand, CDs are unsecured, and the risk factor is directly related to the bank's operations. There is usually a penalty associated with early withdrawals; this limits the short-term flexibility of funds held in CDs. If funds become available that will not be subject to early withdrawal risks, however, CDs provide a sound investment instrument with rates varying with market conditions.

Treasury bills are short-term notes issued by the federal government. While specific amounts of time and interest are stipulated, treasury bills are traded on the open market, thereby increasing their liquidity above that of CDs. The risk is negligible due to the government's backing. Treasury bill rates, therefore, trend slightly lower than CD rates.

Repurchase agreements or repos are bank-related and provide flexible short-term investment opportunities. They are generally pools of funds that are backed by treasury bills. Odd lots are available, and terms may be for as short a period as one day. Repo rates are generally lower than for treasury bills, due to the bank's operating percentage.

Savings accounts are common vehicles used for individual savings. Amounts in such accounts are flexible and liquid and are insured to a specified level. Interest rates on savings accounts are the lowest of any of the rates cited above.

Hospital administrators should discuss particular investment plans and available instruments with several sources, including a number of banks, to ensure the maximum return for the risk assumed and the most favorable banking relationships.

COMMUNITY MEDICAL CENTER: WORKING CAPITAL MANAGEMENT

Based on the historic financial statements presented in previous chapters, the reader, as president of Community Medical Center, is now in a position to evaluate the working capital management of the center and to establish policies for future operations. As a starting point, the various aspects of working capital should be examined in the light of operating results, and objective goals should be established for cash and payables management. The reader should bear in mind that the results of this analysis will heavily influence future operations with regard to liquidity and overall working capital management. The following steps are involved in the analysis:

• List key relationships relative to working capital and operations.

- Subjectively evaluate past management and identify important future trends.

- List specific, objective goals relative to the management of working capital at Community Medical Center.

Chapter 10

Maximizing Reimbursement

INTRODUCTION

As noted in Chapter 4, cost reimbursement is the basis for a growing percentage of hospital activity. The hospital's administration must accordingly be continuously aware of areas that will maximize reimbursement and of the impact on reimbursement of various managerial actions such as rate setting. When a difference in interpretation of regulations occurs between the hospital and Medicare, various appeal mechanisms are available to the hospital, including the court system. An issue that should be carefully reviewed by a hospital's administration is the maximization of reimbursement through the appeal process.

MEDICARE UTILIZATION AND RATE SETTING

An example of a Medicare cost and utilization summary that is useful in determining criteria for potential cost center isolation and alternative charge structures is shown in Table 10–1.

Table 10–1 Analysis of Cost to Charge and Medicare Utilization Ratios

Area	Cost to Charge	Medicare Utilization	Total Chgs	Medicare
Operating room	.929004	$166,390	$1,054,906	15.773
Recovery room	.573610	19,789	148,540	13.322
Delivery and labor	1.837440	-0-	103,278	-0-
Anesthesia	.390322	63,873	586,331	10.894
Radiology	.530585	273,549	1,622,403	16.861
Laboratory	.513820	603,089	1,967,576	30.650

Table 10–1 continued

Blood	.767249	41,700	139,497	29.893
Oxygen therapy	.763844	349,555	659,242	53.024
Physical therapy	1.175430	38,099	168,190	22.652
Occupational therapy	6.033290	1,605	4,626	34.695
EKG	.298950	129,955	370,938	35.034
EEG	.431223	11,647	88,045	13.228
Medical supplies	.797346	210,208	337,941	62.202
Drugs	.551108	461,976	1,201,484	38.450
Emergency room	.890885	41,271	593,970	0.0695

Routine per diem $68.05765
ICU per diem $158.08653

Routine and intensive care unit (ICU) areas are reimbursed via a per diem computation; therefore, a percentage of Medicare utilization in these areas may be computed on a Medicare days/total days basis. For 1978, this computation yields a Medicare percentage of 28.517 in routine and 53.218 in ICU.

From a managerial viewpoint, the data in Table 10–1 provides the information necessary for a data flow analysis of the Medicare cost report. In analyzing cost-finding alternatives, the highest costs possible should be allocated to those areas with the highest Medicare utilization, for example, medical supplies with a 62 percent Medicare utilization rate or ICU with a 53 percent Medicare utilization rate.

Various statistics for performing the step-down should be utilized. Alternative bases acceptable to Medicare should be explored and evaluated. In addition to analyzing alternative step-down bases, the hospital should analyze its chart of accounts and the contents of each cost center for potential costs that could be directly allocated before step-down to particularly high utilization areas. An example would be orderly services, which performs functions for ICU and routine areas. Unless a split is made in this area, all costs would be allocated to routine care with a 28.51 percent utilization rate rather than a portion of the costs allocated to ICU with a 53 percent Medicare utilization rate. By becoming familiar with the detailed accounting recording system, the hospital administration will be able to match revenues and full expenses with the most advantageous results in terms of cost reimbursement.

By further analyzing revenues on a procedure-by-procedure basis, highly utilized tests can be identified. Once identified, increased charges for these tests will result in a higher Medicare percentage of utilization in the department. This practice is particularly useful in high cost/charge ratio areas such as physical therapy, operating room, and emergency room. This analysis could result in lower allowance figures. Rates should be the same to all payers for a particular procedure. However, after rates are established, an increase in highly utilized procedures in a particular department can increase reimbursement somewhat.

The second analysis is that of segregation of cost centers for cost reporting. The analysis of Medicare utilization on a procedure-by-procedure basis requires that a detailed log be kept of Medicare activity in each subdepartment. This procedure requires a substantial amount of time in data gathering. Potential benefits must be weighed against cost commitments. Similarly, if a particular cost center is contained in a larger department, for example, intravenous (IV) therapy in pharmacy, it may be advantageous to segregate the area. This segregation is beneficial if the cost-to-charge ratio is substantially different from that in the larger department. The same benefit may be experienced if Medicare utilization of the subdepartment is different from that of the main center. As an example, suppose that IV therapy is in the pharmacy area and the following information is available for the IV therapy area:

Cost	Charges	Ratio	Medicare Charges
$200,000	$190,000	1.05263	$95,000

By segregating the areas, we have the following reimbursement effect:

	Cost	Charges	Ratio	Medicare Charges	Reimbursement
Drugs	$462,147	$1,011,484	.4569	$366,976	$167,671
IV therapy	$200,000	$ 190,000	1.05263	$ 95,000	$100,000
				Total reimbursement	$267,671

Comparison of the $267,671 recomputed reimbursement with the original cost report amount of $254,598 illustrates the benefits of such a segregation.

EFFECTIVE ACCOUNTING POLICIES

The Medicare program reimburses the "full" cost of providing care to its beneficiaries. In many respects, cost is determined by the accounting procedures that are utilized. Optimum benefits are derived from noncash outflow increases in reimbursable costs. The following accounting procedures may be used.

As noted previously, last-in-first-out (LIFO) costing of inventories results in higher operating expenses during periods of inflation. The recent increases in price levels have produced a considerable divergence between LIFO and FIFO pricing methods.

Vacation pay generally accrues to the individual employee in the form of termination pay. Specifically, upon termination, the individual receives the accrued vacation pay. Such a policy results in a modified form of a vested benefit to the individual. As a vested benefit, it is appropriate for the hospital to establish an accrued liability in the amount of the accrued vacation hours multiplied by the vacation pay rate at the end of the fiscal period. Again, expense here has been incurred, resulting in increased cost reimbursement without a direct, immediate cash disbursement.

Directly related to the cost report, there are nonreimbursable costs and revenues which must be offset against total costs to arrive at allowable costs. Examples are cafeteria revenues, physician office costs, parking lot revenues, costs related to convents and the maintenance of religious personnel, costs of patient telephones and television sets, and costs of coffee and gift shops operated by auxiliary personnel. It is imperative that the hospital's accounting system identify costs and revenues on as accurate a basis as possible so as to reduce reliance on an "arbitrary" cost allocation process.

With respect to accounting procedures related to the use of alternative depreciation methods and the timing of the start of depreciation of an asset, while Medicare now requires the use of straight-line depreciation, the hospital may decide on the timing of the beginning of the depreciation. There are several alternative timing procedures, including depreciation on the year-after acquisition, month-by-month depreciation, and one-half year in the year of acquisition. The most accurate timing policy is that of month by month, however, the cost of such a system must be weighed against the benefits in accuracy. Both the month-by-month and the one-half year method accelerate depreciation timing, compared to the year-after-acquisition method.

The above discussion pinpoints the several areas that should be analyzed for potential benefits via the Medicare cost report through the hospital's routine accounting system. Again, it is important that the administration of the hospital evaluate the accounting flows related to the overall operations of the institution. An increase in expense for the purpose of maximizing reimbursement has associated risks in the form of a reduction in net income on the statement of revenues and expenses. The hospital's board should be familiar with the cost reporting procedures in order to put such increased costs into their proper perspective.

Similarly, the hospital's administrators should be aware of the risks involved in planning a sizable bond issue or incurrence of debt. Rating and financial reviews associated with debt require sound revenue-generation trends. A change in accounting procedures to increase expenses to maximize reimbursement could result in a more adverse reaction from bond-rating agencies and the bond market than would be justified by the benefits derived from maximizing reimbursement.

CURRENT MEDICARE ISSUES

Today's hospital environment has given rise to operations and accounting theories that have resulted in unique and controversial interpretations of the Medicare law and regulations. The different methodologies and theories have at times led to conflicts over the interpretation of Medicare regulations. Current areas of interest related to Medicare reimbursement include the following:

- interest income and expense during construction, the handling of specific bond funds, and the relationship of debt to funded depreciation

- limitation on malpractice trust reimbursement to the extent of program claims paid

- costs of special-care units

- costs of related organizations

When a hospital undertakes a major construction program, it is not uncommon for it to incur debt with related interest expense and interest income on unexpended bond funds. Particularly in relation to tax-exempt financing, several funds may be established and held by the independent trustee to ensure payment of the debt service, construction costs, and interest during construction. Usually, these funds are deposited and held by an independent trustee, with the hospital having no control over the funds or over the income from the investment of the funds.

At the present time, Medicare regulations allow the following treatments of funded depreciation and bond funds expense and income:

- Income derived from funded depreciation does not have to be offset against operating interest expense. Funded depreciation is limited to the amount of accumulated depreciation.

- Funded depreciation must be reduced to a zero balance before any debt is incurred for capital acquisitions.

- Interest expense and income during construction must be capitalized. The income on unexpended bond funds is to be offset only to the extent of the interest expense that is capitalized.

The operating and reimbursement ramifications of these regulations are profound. First, it is very difficult to reduce funded depreciation to a zero balance. The result of not totally depleting the funded depreciation account to zero is a required offset of interest income on the funds held at the time of the borrowing until the funds have been spent for capital acquisitions on a FIFO basis. The funded depreciation account is segregated. Therefore, expenditures are measured by withdrawals from funded depreciation and expended for capital acquisitions.

Amounts borrowed to establish specific indentured, trusteed funds, such as a debt service reserve fund, are usually held for the life of the bond issue. The income from these funds, whether or not under the control of the hospital, must be offset against expense. A valid argument for not offsetting fund revenues is that these funds are established from funded depreciation and the income is treated as funded depreciation with no offset of the revenue.

Finally, the proper treatment of interest expense during construction is still being debated. Whether to capitalize or expense interest during construction is a controversial subject in the accounting profession, even though Medicare requires capitalization.

The hospital must not lose sight of Medicare ramifications in the decision to incur debt. Careful planning related to funded depreciation and the structuring of required funds through the indenture could avoid numerous reimbursement adjustments that may not have been adequately taken into account in the financing decision process.

During the period of dramatic inflation in malpractice insurance premiums, many hospitals established self-insurance trusts and undertook risk-management programs. The funding levels of the trusts were based on actuarial studies on a hospital-by-hospital basis. Hospitals were therefore able to avoid costly insurance premiums and to establish funds that were reasonably based on each hospital's long-range experience. Medicare regulations responded accordingly and allowed reimbursement for funds deposited with an independent trustee in amounts based on current actuarial studies combined with a risk-management program. More recently, Medicare has proposed that only that proportion of funding that represents the percentage of historic Medicare settlements of total malpractice settlements be allowed. If experience does not yield a reasonable volume of base data, a national average of as low as 5 percent would be utilized. This would have a direct impact on reimbursement, as illustrated in the following example.

Assume that actuarial findings indicate a funding level of $460,000 and that the Medicare average utilization rate is 30 percent. In this case, the previous reimbursement would be .30 × $460,000 = $138,000. Under the new proposal, the reimbursement may be only .05 × $460,000 = $23,000. The difference in reimbursement is about $115,000.

There will probably be appeals from this regulation, based on the argument that a distinction by class of payer is impossible for a normal operating cost such as malpractice funding. Hospital administrators should be aware of the trend indicated by this proposal so that alternative plans may be instituted to recoup the loss of reimbursement.

We have previously mentioned the benefits of segmenting various cost centers of the hospital. Special-care areas, such as physical and respiratory rehabilitation units, usually have higher costs and higher levels of Medicare activity. In some instances, efforts have been made to segment routine care into special care areas. However, Medicare regulations require that six conditions be met before a special care area is established:

1. The unit must be in a hospital.
2. The care required must be extraordinary.
3. The care in the unit must be concentrated.
4. The care in the unit must be continuous.
5. The unit must be physically identifiable as separate from general patient-care areas.
6. The unit must have specific, written policies.

These criteria require a great deal of interpretation of what is "extraordinary," "concentrated," "continuous," and so on. Therefore, a hospital should analyze the proposed segmented area and obtain advance approval from the Medicare intermediary for the unit.

Finally, Medicare regulations on reimbursement provide for reimbursement of patient-related costs that are reasonable in amount and would be incurred by a prudent buyer. Medicare regulations have specifically addressed acquisitions from related organizations and have limited costs to the original acquisition cost, in the light of a reasonableness test of comparable goods available in the market. In principle, costs applicable to services, facilities, and supplies furnished to the provider by organizations related to the provider by common ownership or control are includable in the allowable cost to the related organization. However, such costs must not exceed the price of comparable services, facilities, or supplies that could be purchased elsewhere. As defined, common ownership exists when an individual possesses significant ownership or equity in the provider and in the institution or organization servicing the provider and when that individual also has the power, directly or indirectly, significantly to influence or direct the actions or policies of the organization or institution.

The above regulations provide for a substantial amount of individual interpretation as to ownership, control, and reasonable definitions. Their implications are far-reaching, as hospitals look for other business income, form multiinstitutional systems, and incur management contracts.

APPEAL PROCEDURES

As the reader has probably deduced, Medicare regulations do not always provide methods that apply in all circumstances or allow for alternative interpretations of the law and regulations. To alleviate this situation, the 1972 Medicare Act (P.L. 92–603) established the Provider Reimbursement Review Board (PRRB) under the secretary of HHS to hear provider complaints concerning intermediaries' determinations of reimbursement. The five members of the PRRB include two representatives of providers; the remaining three must be knowledgeable of cost reimbursement and at least one must be a certified public accountant. The board's actions must be in accordance with the statutory provisions of the Medicare Act (Title XVIII) and associated regulations. All rulings of the PRRB are subject to review by the secretary of HHS, as delegated to the administrator of the Health Care Financing Administration (HCFA), which is a part of HHS. A decision of the board is final unless the secretary reverses, affirms, or modifies the board's decision within 60 days after the provider is notified of the decision. A flow chart of the PRRB process is shown in Figure 10–1.

If the provider is not satisfied with the ruling of the PRRB or the HCFA administrator, the provider may seek judicial review of the board decision. The suit must be filed in the provider's local federal district court or in the District of Columbia. The final decision by the HCFA administrator becomes the basis for the appeal, and the appeal must be filed within 60 days after the administrator's notification of the decision.

In the judicial review process, no new evidence is allowed to be introduced beyond the documentation related to the PRRB process. Therefore, it is imperative that all facts and documentation be presented at the PRRB level in anticipation that a judicial review will be necessary. If the provider's case is sound, either on the specific issues or on the principles contained in the regulations, the provider should individually or collectively explore the potential of the case with competent consultants. In this way, the use of the provider appeal procedures can aid in identifying those reimbursement regulations that should apply in the case.

Figure 10–1 Summary Time Chart of the Medicare Appeal Process

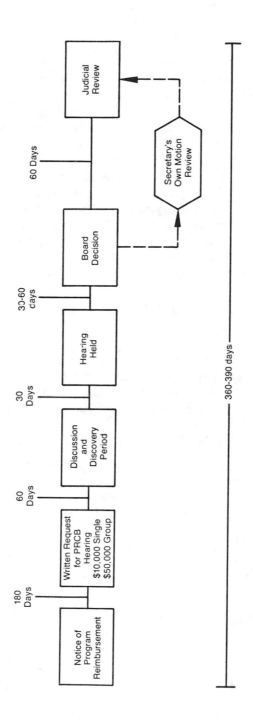

SUMMARY

To put the above discussion in proper perspective, it should be emphasized that routine cost limitations must be considered when determining the most advantageous method of managing cost reimbursement programs. Increasing cost in a particular area may result in the hospital's exceeding such cost limits. Also, it must be remembered that the Medicare program reimburses the lower of costs or charges. Therefore, the provider must be aware of the relationship of cost to charges in the cost reporting and rate setting process.

Finally, it should be noted that the Medicare program has a very active fraud and abuse monitoring program. A hospital must not fraudulently present a statement of cost for payment because of altered statistics. If the hospital takes a different view, it should disclose this in the submission of the cost report to the Medicare program. The hospital must continuously maintain its research facilities and be in constant communication with Medicare and the intermediary regarding regulations, laws, and interpretations.

COMMUNITY MEDICAL CENTER: MAXIMIZING REIMBURSEMENT

The reader may assume that the cost/charge ratios and percentages presented in Table 10–1 apply to the Medicare activity for Community Medical Center for 1978. To develop a rate structure policy for the center to maximize reimbursement, the reader should address the following questions:

- What general steps should be taken in the development of a maximization rate structure?

- From the data presented, which areas should be emphasized in the development of the revised charge structure?

- Assuming that the blood gas analysis test in respiratory (oxygen) therapy has a Medicare utilization rate of 70 percent and the present charge is $80 per test with 3,000 analyses done each year, what is the reimbursement effect of increasing the charge for this test to $120 per analysis?

The major expansion program that the medical center is contemplating could entail a substantial bond issue, including the refinancing of existing debt and necessary construction funds. As president of Community Medical Center, the reader must develop a financing strategy that minimizes any adverse Medicare reimbursement effects taking into consideration the following:

- Funded depreciation should be zero at the time of financing. What are the financing implications of this requirement?

- Bond funds have common financing elements related to construction and current expense, for example, refinancing debt and debt service reserve funds. What steps should be taken regarding the offset of interest income or the use of funded depreciation to establish the bond-related funds of debt service reserve, interest during construction, and flotation costs?

Chapter 11

Capital Asset Evaluation and Long-Term Financing

INTRODUCTION

Public Law 93–641, commonly known as the Comprehensive Health Planning Act, established a framework for the evaluation of capital acquisitions on a local and state level. At the local level where the preliminary need and economic feasibility of a project are evaluated, the act established the Health Systems Agencies (HSAs). At the state level, certificate of need legislation was mandated, providing for Health Facilities Planning Boards to evaluate projects and determine the final approval or disapproval of the reviewable projects. These systems require that individual hospitals and health services evaluate proposed projects on a systematic basis. Such an analysis requires detailed revenue and expense projections, identification of financing requirements, and exploration of alternative financing and delivery methods.

CAPITAL EXPENDITURE EVALUATION

Health care institutions have historically fallen behind other industries in evaluating major capital expenditures. During the period when Hill-Burton funds were readily available, health care construction skyrocketed. Lending institutions were rather lax in requiring detailed feasibility studies in health care institutions due to the relatively low risk associated with a non-price-regulated industry. Recently, health care facilities in particular are facing tighter controls on capital expenditures through enactment of various sections of P.L. 92–603 and P.L. 93–641. Hospitals are facing state planning boards and area planning agencies in their quest for approval to build or acquire capital items. Lending institutions will continue to be pressed by all industries for funds, with the federal government also trying to finance its deficit spending.

Thus, health care facilities will be faced with a restrictive, critical environment when they attempt capital expenditures. This environment will force providers to evaluate health care expenditures more critically.

In this section, we will deal with the specifics and technical aspects of three common methods of capital expenditure evaluation—payback, net present value, and internal rate of return—and will attempt to analyze each technique with an eye towards meaningfulness and ease of implementation.

Payback

The payback method of evaluating capital expenditures began and grew with conservative financial management styles. It is a method by which management can rationalize how "safe" its investments are by seeing how fast revenues generated from an investment accumulate to exceed the original payout. The period up to the point where the sum of revenues equals original investment is know as the payback period. We thus have PP = I/R, where PP = payback period, I = original investment, and R = net revenues associated with the investment.

Benefits of this method are ease of application and an inherent ranking system in which the shorter the payback period, the better the investment. However, one does not have to think very hard to see major flaws in this method. For example, which is the "better" investment in the following case: A "costs" $1,000,000, and B "costs" $1,000,000. A's revenue life is one year, generating $1,000,000 the first year; B generates $500,000 for 20 years. PP for A is one year, and for B, two years. In deciding which is the better investment, it should be noted that the payback method does not recognize revenues beyond the payback period and does not take into account the time value of money.

Net Present Value

The net present value (NPV) method of evaluating capital expenditures takes into account revenues during the entire useful life of the investment and also the time value of money. The basis of a present value analysis is the question, "Would you rather have $1 now or $1 a year from now?" Obviously, you would rather have $1 now because it could be invested in a five-percent savings account and be "worth" $1.05 a year from now. Conversely, a $1 returned a year from now, assuming a required or available return of five percent, is worth $1/$1.05 or $0.952 now. Therefore, you would lend $.952 at five percent to get $1 back in a year. For two years, you would lend $1/$1.05^2 at five percent or $.907 to get back $1 two years from now.

We are thus led to a general rule: To find the present value (PV) of an investment returning $1 after n years at r interest we have $PV = \$1/(1 + r)^n$. What does this mean? Assume a piece of laboratory equipment costs $20,000 with a useful life of five years, the estimated salvage value at the end of five years is $1,000, and net cash inflows from operations are as follows:

	Year				
	1	2	3	4	5
Cash	$5,000	$3,000	$4,000	$5,000	$6,000
Salvage					1,000
Total Cash inflows	$5,000	$3,000	$4,000	$5,000	$7,000

To arrive at the net cash inflows, we took into account the incremental cash generated from the equipment and the incremental cash expenditures due to the equipment. Because we are dealing with cash flows throughout the analysis, we do not use accrual accounting.

The facility needs to establish an interest rate to be used in the analysis. To do this, a reasonable estimate is the average weighted cost of capital for outstanding debt or available investment returns on cash investments for each of the future years. The higher rate is the more conservative for purposes of this analysis.

Assume that in our example the facility requires a seven-percent return on its investment. We can thus formulate the tableau shown in Table 11–1. From this we can see that the present value of the cash outlays exceeded the present values of the cash inflows with the required seven-percent "hurdle rate." The facility would have been "better-off" investing the $20,000 in a seven-percent savings account. Net present value analysis takes into account the timing, amounts, and discount factors over the life of the investment project. Conversely, we could have worked backwards, developing an internal rate of return for the project by finding the discount rate that would make the net present value of the project zero. A comparison could thus be made of the internal rate of return with the hurdle rate necessary to be achieved to make the project "worthwhile" to the institution.

Internal Rate of Return

The third technique is that of internal rate of return, a method very similar to that of net present value. A simple definition of the internal rate of return is that discount rate that will yield a net present value of zero for the project or acquisition. In the previous example, the ($637) net present value of the laboratory equipment is close to zero; therefore, the internal rate of return is slightly less than the seven percent used in the analysis. The actual

Table 11-1 Formulation of Net Present Value

Description \ Period	NOW	Year 1	Year 2	Year 3	Year 4	Year 5
Cash out	$20,000					
Cash in operations		$5,000	$3,000	$4,000	$5,000	$6,000
Salvage						1,000
Net cash in (out) ①	(20,000)	5,000	3,000	4,000	5,000	7,000
PV factor	$\frac{1}{(1+.07)^0}$	$\frac{1}{(1+.07)^1}$	$\frac{1}{(1+.07)^2}$	$\frac{1}{(1+.07)^3}$	$\frac{1}{(1+.07)^4}$	$\frac{1}{(1+.07)^5}$
②	1	.9345	.8734	.8163	.7629	.7130
① × ② = ③ Present Value	($20,000)	$4,673	$2,620	$3,265	$3,814	$4,991

internal rate of return of the laboratory equipment is 5.99 percent, which is derived by trial and error for various discount rates. If the initial factor yields a positive net present value, the discount factor must be increased on the next iteration. Similarly, as in the above example, a negative net present value requires a reduction in the discount factor on the next attempt. The result of the use of the internal rate of return is the same as that for net present value. The higher the internal rate of return, the more favorable the project. Consequently, projects may be ranked by internal rate of return. Also, the hospital may want to establish a minimum "hurdle" rate for projects. In this case, a project would be required to have an internal rate of return above a set minimum before it would be given further consideration.

PRESENT-VALUE CONSIDERATIONS OF ANNUITIES

The general format for the computation of discounted cash flows (DCF) is:

$$DCF = \sum_{i=1}^{n} (1/(1+r)^i) \times CF_i$$

where: n is the time period,
r is the discount factor, and
CF is the cash flow for the period

If cash flows for equal time periods were equal, the general formula would be simplified to:

$$DCF = CF \sum_{i=1}^{n} 1/(1 + r)^i$$

where CF is constant

Whenever the cash flow is the same for equally spaced time periods, it is said to be an annuity, and the computation

$$CF \sum_{i=1}^{n} 1/(1 + r)^i$$

is known as the present value of the annuity and

$$\sum_{i=1}^{n} 1/(1 + r)^i$$

is the discount factor for the annuity. If cash flows are the same for each year, the discounted cash flow is easily computed by a simple multiplication procedure. When the problem is the determination of the internal rate of return for a capital acquisition/period,

$$CF = \sum_{i=1}^{n} 1/(1 + r)^i$$

The task now is one of determining which discount rate solves the above equation. This procedure is simplified by the use of tables which have computed

$$\sum_{i=1}^{n} 1/(1 + r)^i$$

for various time periods and discount factors. The form

$$\sum_{i=1}^{n} 1/(1 + r)^i$$

is a geometric progression that equals $(1 - (1 + r)^{-n})/r$ and the limit of which, as n approaches infinity, is $1/r$. To determine the internal rate of return of an annuity, suppose that the laboratory equipment cited above cost $20,000 and had a life of five years and an annual cash flow of +$5276. The discount factor for the internal rate of return is determined by the following formula:

$$\text{Purchase price/Period cash flow} = \sum_{i=1}^{n} 1/(1 + r)^i \text{ or } \$20,000/\$5,276 = 3.7907$$

We find the number 3.7907 for five years is the corresponding discount factor of 10 percent. Therefore, the internal rate of return is 10 percent.

In its general format, a lease is a form of annuity with equal payments over evenly spaced time periods, with or without lump-sum payments at the end of the lease. The effective rate of the lease may be computed by determining the discount rate that will discount the future cash payments to the current purchase price of the leased item.

Suppose that a hospital leases a group of equipment items costing $385,082 for 10 years, with an annual payment of $60,000 for each of the 10 years and a payment of $100,000 at the end of the lease (the $100,000 being the fair market value of the equipment at the end of the lease). By utilizing trial and error, one may determine the discount rate of 11 percent for the lease as follows. The value of an annuity for 10 years at 11 percent is 5.8892. The percent value of a $1 paid at the end of the 11th year at 11 percent is .3173. By applying these factors to the above example, we have the following present value of the lease payments: (5.8892)($60,000) + (.3173)($100,000) = $353,354 + $31,728 = $385,082, which is the current purchase price of the equipment.

This example illustrates a "true" or operating lease under the definition of FAS–13 as described earlier. Suppose that a lease arrangement provides for ten annual payments of $50,000 for a piece of equipment with a current cost of $307,228, with the title passing to the hospital at the end of the lease. Under FAS–13, this is a capital lease. The interest rate associated with the lease is computed as follows: The discount factor is $307,228/$50,000 = 6.14456. Consequently, the transaction entries to establish the capital lease would be:

	Debit	Credit
Capital Asset	$307,228	
Debt		$307,228

Each year when the $50,000 payment is made, interest on the outstanding balance (.10 × current principal) is computed and booked along with depreciation on the $307,228. Therefore, in the first year, depreciation is $307,228/10 = $30,722, and interest is $307,228 × .10 = $30,722, for a total expense of $61,444. In this case, the allowable expense is greater than the $50,000 lease payment in the early years of the lease and becomes less as the principal and therefore interest are reduced.

In the financial evaluation of capital asset acquisitions or individual operational programs, it is necessary to evaluate all cash flows of the operation over the useful life of the program. Consequently, a review of the integral components of a cash flow analysis is appropriate at this point.

As noted earlier, the general format for a statement of cash flow is:

Gross revenue	$xxx,xxx
Gross expenses	(yyy,yyy)
Depreciation	(zzz,zzz)
	(1)
(1) × Medicare %	(aaa,aaa)
Depreciation	zzz,zzz
Bad debts	(bbb,bbb)
Other % × Gross revenue	ccc,ccc
	Cash Flow

The factor ccc,ccc in the above format represents the change in items in other areas of the noncash balance sheet that should remain relatively constant for incremental activity over a period of time. This excludes capital requirements directly related to the project under evaluation and discrete, identifiable items such as increased receivables.

The "Other Revenue/Expense" component, which should be monitored administratively, will be held as a constant percentage factor in the discussion to follow. This component may be developed by trending period cash flows, excluding operations and capital acquisitions, as a percentage of gross revenues with significant and expected variances reflected in project cash flows. When evaluating a project, only incremental cash flow is relevant to the decision. Therefore, both direct increases and decreases in revenues and expenses should be reflected in the analysis. Also, note that depreciation is a cash flow item only in reference to Medicare reimbursement.

FINANCING ALTERNATIVES FOR A MAJOR EQUIPMENT PURCHASE

The method of financing has a direct relationship to project cash flow, as illustrated in the following example. Suppose the hospital anticipates the acquisition of a CAT scanner in the radiology department. Salaries are expected to increase $16,000, supplies will increase $2,000, and other expenses will increase $8,000 per year. Revenues are based on a $230 charge per procedure for 1,000 expected procedures per year. It is expected that there will be no reduction in other procedures performed in the hospital. The cost of the equipment is $500,000 with a useful life of seven years. Historically, 4 percent of gross charges are bad debts, and there is a 52 percent third party payer utilization cost. Available financing methods include leasing the equipment for five years with a purchase option of $143,000 at the end of the fifth year and an annual lease payment of $71,614. The hospital could borrow $400,000 at nine percent interest for seven years. The hospital could purchase the equipment directly from funded depreciation.

The hospital must now determine the appropriate discount rate above which the project becomes feasible. This step is necessary whether present-value or internal-rate-of-return techniques are utilized. The determination of the appropriate "hurdle" rate is dependent on the availability of funds, the rate of return obtainable from general investments, and the price rises inherent in the project both from usage and from future inflation.

Generally, the rate of interest obtainable on investments in instruments such as certificates of deposit is a good starting point for rate determination. Added to this rate is a factor for internally determined allocation restrictions. Finally, a factor for risk is built into the rate. As an example, suppose that the hospital could invest in certificates of deposit that yield eight percent. Also, due to the fact that all projects earning eight percent may not be financed, the hospital requires a two-percent add-on for projects to be considered.

Finally, the hospital requires a varying rate addition depending on the following schedule of requirements:

- If the project is industry-wide and generally accepted, the risk is minimal and a 1-percent addition is required. If not, a 4-percent addition is made.

- If the project costs are 10 percent or less of funded depreciation, a 1-percent add-on is required. From 11 to 20 percent, the add-on is 2 percent; from 21 to 50 percent, 3 percent; from 51 to 70 percent, 4 percent; from 71 to 90 percent, 5 percent; and from 91 to 100 percent, 6 percent.

- If the project is required by law or is essential for survival, no addition is required.

While somewhat arbitrary, this schedule does quantify the subjective evaluation of risk. The relationship of these criteria to the CAT scanner project yields the following hurdle rate: investment (8%) + criteria (2%) + risk acceptance (1%) + risk cost (1%) = 12 percent.

In addition to being concerned with internal feasibility, the hospital must comply with the planning legislation in the state as required by P.L. 93–641. The procedural flow related to the certificate of need begins with the HSA. The criteria used in the project review deal with need and financial feasibility. It must be demonstrated that the reviewed project is a medical necessity for the population serviced by the institution, that the project does not represent a duplication of services, and that there is community and physician support for the hospital and project. It is essential that, for each reviewable project, the hospital research the possibility of sharing of services and incorporate the results into a financial feasibility alternative for the project. Such area-wide planning is basic to the intent of the law that an increase in shared services should result in an increase in area-wide delivery efficiency and consequently a reduction in overall costs.

In the case of the CAT scanner, the hospital must identify alternative delivery modes, whether on a shared basis with area institutions or through the use of alternative treatment vehicles. Therefore, a complete evaluation of the CAT project would include modality comparisons of the CAT with ultrasound and normal x-ray treatments, nuclear medicine procedures, and even the use of exploratory surgery. The most difficult question to address is that concerning the cost/benefit of saving lives. There is no single value for a future benefit of a lifesaving treatment. Subjectively, however, one might conclude that a project is merely a convenience, not a necessity, particularly if there is a similar program in the immediate area.

In the financial evaluation of the CAT scanner program, it is necessary to begin with a determination of the cash flow associated with each financing alternative. In summary, we have the following cash flow data: procedures, 1,000; charge per procedure, $230; salaries, $16,000; supplies, $2,000; other, $8,000; life, 7 years; cost, $500,000; internal rate of return required, 12 percent; bad debts, 4 percent; and contractual allowances, 52 percent. The three financing alternatives are:

1. Lease (operating): Cash outflow is $71,614 for five years, with purchase for $143,000 at the end of the fifth year. No salvage value is assumed.
2. Borrow: Borrow $500,000 at nine percent interest for seven years.
3. Finance internally: Cash outflow is $500,000 initially.

Lease

For the lease (operating) alternative, the relevant data are presented in Tables 11–2 and 11–3. The discount factor associated with an annuity for four years at 12 percent is 3.0373. The discount factor from Table 11–4 for Year 5 at 12 percent is .56743, and the discount factors for Years 6 and 7 are .50663 and .4523 respectively. Discounting the cash flows results in the following:

Years 1 to 4 ($54,345 × 3.0373)	$165,062
Year 5 ($88,655 × .56743)	(50,305)
Years 6 and 7 ($148,520 × (.50663 = .4523)	142,416
Net present value	$257,173

Table 11–2 Cash Flow Computation

For years 1 to 5:

Gross revenue (1,000 × $230)	$230,000
Salaries	(16,000)
Supplies	(2,000)
Other	(8,000)
Leasing	(71,614)
	$132,386
	× .52
Contractual allowances	$ 68,841
Bad debts ($230,000 × .04)	$ 9,200

For years 6 and 7:

Gross revenue	$230,000
Salaries	(16,000)
Supplies	(2,000)
Other	(8,000)
Depreciation (143,000/2)	(115,000)
	$ 89,000
	× .52
Contractual allowances	$ 46,280
Bad Debts ($230,000 × .04)	$ 9,200

Table 11-3 Statement of Cash Flow

	Years 1–4	Year 5	Years 6 & 7
Gross revenue	$230,000	$230,000	$230,000
Increased expenses			
Salaries	(16,000)	(16,000)	(16,000)
Supplies	(2,000)	(2,000)	(2,000)
Other	(8,000)	(8,000)	(8,000)
Leasing	(71,614)	(71,614)	-0-
Bad debts	(9,200)	(9,200)	(9,200)
Contractual allowances	(68,841)	(68,841)	(46,280)
Equipment cost		(143,000)	
Net Cash Flow	$ 54,345	$(88,655)	$148,520

Borrow

If $500,000 is borrowed for seven years, at 9 percent interest, the first task is to determine annual debt service. In effect, future cash flow payments for principle and interest on incurred debt at a particular rate of interest may be defined as those cash payments discounted at the interest rate equal to the principle borrowed. In this case, we have an annuity situation where the following formula must be solved:

$$\text{Principle} / \sum_{i=1}^{n} 1/(1 + r)^i = \text{Cash flow debt service.}$$

$$\text{Here, } \$500,000 / \sum_{i=1}^{7} 1/(1 + .09)^7 = \text{Cash flow debt service.}$$

$$\text{From Table 11–3 we know } \sum_{i=1}^{7} 1/(1.09)^7 = 5.0330.$$

Therefore, annual debt service is $500,000/5.0330 = $99,344. In this case, we have both depreciation and interest. Depreciation is $500,000/7 =

$71,428 on a straight-line basis. Interest is nine percent of the outstanding balance as outlined in the following table:

Year	Outstanding Balance	Interest	Debt Service	Principle
1	$500,000	$45,000	$99,344	$54,344
2	445,656	40,109	99,344	59,235
3	386,421	34,778	99,344	64,566
4	321,855	28,967	99,344	70,377
5	251,478	22,633	99,344	76,711
6	174,767	15,729	99,344	83,615
7	91,152	8,203	99,344	91,140

Therefore, the annual cash flows are as indicated in Table 11–4. The sum of the discounted cash flows is the net present value of $193,735.

Finance Internally

The use of internal funded depreciation results in direct acquisition of the asset. However, there is an imputed cost of using invested funds that is

---

Table 11-4 Annual Cash Flows

Year	1	2	3	4	5	6	7
Gross revenue	$230,000	$230,000	$230,000	$230,000	$230,000	$230,000	$230,000
Salaries	(16,000)	(16,000)	(16,000)	(16,000)	(16,000)	(16,000)	(16,000)
Supplies	(2,000)	(2,000)	(2,000)	(2,000)	(2,000)	(2,000)	(2,000)
Other	(8,000)	(8,000)	(8,000)	(8,000)	(8,000)	(8,000)	(8,000)
Debt service	(99,344)	(99,344)	(99,344)	(99,344)	(99,344)	(99,344)	(99,344)
Contingency allowance	(45,537)	(48,081)	(50,853)	(53,875)	(57,168)	(60,578)	(64,672)
Bad debts	(9,200)	(9,200)	(9,200)	(9,200)	(9,200)	(9,000)	(9,000)
Net cash flow	49,919	47,375	44,603	41,581	38,288	34,698	30,784
Discount Factor	.8928	.7972	.7118	.6355	.5674	.5066	.4523
Discounted cash flow	$ 44,568	$ 37,767	$ 31,748	$ 26,425	$ 21,725	$ 17,578	$ 13,924

directly reflected in the discount rate. In this financing alternative, we have the following cash flows:

Year 0: ($500,000) as the initial purchase price.
Years 1 to 7:

Gross revenue	$230,000
Salaries	(16,000)
Supplies	(2,000)
Other	(8,000)
Depreciation	(71,428)
	132,572
	× .52
Contractual allowances	(68,937)
Bad debts	(9,200)

Therefore, the annual cash flow is:

Gross revenue	$230,000
Salaries	(16,000)
Supplies	(2,000)
Other	(8,000)
Contractual allowances	(68,937)
Bad debts	(9,200)
Net cash flow	$125,863

At the time of the initial purchase, the formula $1/(1 + i)^n$ for $n = 0$ is equal to 1. For seven years at 12 percent, the discount factor is 4.5638. Therefore, the present value of the annual cash inflow is $125,863 × 4.5638 = $574,414 with a net present value of $574,414 − $500,000 = $74,414.

Summary

Thus, each of the three financing alternatives yields a positive net present value. It is therefore necessary to develop evaluation criteria for selecting the proper alternative. The first criterion could be the selection of the alternative with the highest positive net present value. The net present value of the three alternatives are:

Alternative	Net Present Value
1	$257,173
2	$193,735
3	$ 74,414

Utilizing this criterion, the first alternative, leasing, would be selected.

A second, and probably a more accurate criterion, is a ranking based on the internal rate of return of the projects, as described in an earlier section. The reader should be able to determine the results based on this criterion.

It can now be seen that there are various factors involved in the selection of a financing method. First, as shown in our discussions of Medicare regulations, debt interest expense may not be allowable by Medicare if there are funds available in funded depreciation. Interest income on funded depreciation may have to be offset if debt is incurred. Therefore, the hospital must analyze its particular circumstances in the light of Medicare regulations. It should be remembered that Medicare restrictions may not invalidate a favorable method of financing. There may be unfavorable terms or interest rates associated with leasing or debt. Also, there is the possibility that indenture restrictions may prohibit incurrence of debt or lease arrangements. Similarly, the hospital may want to maintain a more liquid cash position, particularly if interest rates are expected to increase.

In any case, particularly given the historic lack of leverage in the hospital industry, all financing possibilities should be explored. Acquisitions may be made utilizing debt or leases with payments over extended periods of time without immediate depletion of liquid reserves.

EVALUATION OF LONG-TERM FINANCING ALTERNATIVES

As noted in Chapter 5, there are several long-term financing alternatives available to hospitals. Of these, three will be examined here: mortgages, taxable bonds, and tax-exempt bonds.

Mortgages

Assuming mortgage financing by Community Medical Center for its proposed expansion project, interim financing would be required during the estimated three-year construction program. Short-term financing of the magnitude needed would require a firm take-out at the end of the construction program. Also, the financing would require at least a 30 percent contribution by the center. Based on the center's balance sheets, the center could not commit sufficient funds to put into place the required 30 percent of $20,594,000 or $6,178,200. Even though flotation costs are about 1 percent of the amount financed, it does not appear that mortgage financing is a viable alternative for the center.

Taxable Bonds

Taxable bonds would be a viable long-term financing alternative for the center. In this case interim financing would not be required, and flotation costs would be about 2 percent of the amount borrowed. Current rates are about 10.5 percent with a term of about 20 years. Given the minimum construction cost and refinancing of $25,487,402, and assuming a debt financing of 80 percent of construction cost, the minimum debt would be 80 percent of $20,594,000 or $16,475,200, plus the refinancing of $4,893,402, for a total $21,368,602. Assuming that interest during construction for three years is borrowed, the center then has $21,368,602/(1 − (3 × .105)) = $30,656,934 of debt. If financing costs of about 2 percent of the financing amount must be borrowed, the center will have a debt requirement of $32,133,236, with a contribution of 20 percent × $20,594,000 = $4,118,800 required at the beginning or end of the construction program. This amount would come from funded depreciation from internally generated funds.

It is possible to reduce the amount of debt by taking into account the interest earned during construction. If an average rate of 7 percent is expected to be earned on funds during construction, the amount of borrowing would be reduced to about $30,500,000. In effect, a debt of $30,500,000 would be required to finance $25,594,000 worth of construction and refinancing. At 10.5 percent for 20 years, annual debt service would be $3,705,545 or about $3,700,000. The effective rate of interest for this proposed financing alternative is computed as follows: The discount factor = $25,594,000/$3,700,000 = 6.9172. The discount rate associated with 6.9172 for 20 years is about 13.25 percent, which is considerably above the 10.5 percent coupon rate.

Tax-Exempt Bonds

Tax-exempt bonds have become an increasingly viable alternative in long-term debt financing. There are several variations of this method, depending to a significant extent on the state in which the hospital is located. States with "home-rule" provisions in their constitutions do not require title to pass to a municipality. In these states, title to the hospital remains with the hospital via a "pass-through" mortgage where the municipality serves only as the issuing authority. The hospital is solely liable for payment of the debt; no liability is assumed by the municipality. In states without home-rule provisions, title passes to the municipality at the inception of the bond issue. The hospital in effect has a capital lease with the issuing authority. Available issuing agents include municipalities and specially created state financing authorities whose sole purpose is to provide a vehicle for issuing tax-exempt bonds.

While tax-exempt bonds carry a lower rate of interest than taxable bonds or mortgages, they carry several common restrictions that add to the effective financing costs.

In the case of the center's construction project, given financing of $28,500,000 for 30 years, the computation of the effective rate of interest using a $2,296,000 or 7 percent rate is 8.4 percent, which is an even better cost-effective mode of financing.

COMMUNITY MEDICAL CENTER: LONG-TERM FINANCING ALTERNATIVES

The reader should at this point prepare an analysis of the three methods of financing we have presented, including the pros and cons of each method. As president of Community Medical Center, the reader should determine the appropriate initial financial planning point, given the financials in the following feasibility study summary:

Summary of Assumptions in Forecasted Financial Statements

Interest Expense and Long-Term Debt

Interest expense on the proposed center revenue bonds is estimated at 6.75 percent annually. Interest expense related to applicable construction in progress, net of interest income on invested trusteed funds, has been capitalized during the construction period.

Nonoperating Revenue

Forecasted nonoperating revenue consists of estimated interest at five percent per year on invested board-designated and trusteed funds. Interest income on trusteed funds during the construction period is assumed to be offset against capitalized interest expense.

Working Capital

Forecasted working capital components are based on recent center experience and discussions with the center's administration. The major working capital requirements are:

Operating cash	15 days of operating expenses excluding depreciation and interest. Forecasted cash on hand

	in excess of operating cash is included in board-designated funds.
Accounts receivable	62 days of patient revenues
Inventories	14 days of nonsalary expenses, excluding depreciation and interest
Prepaid expenses	1.5 days of nonsalary expenses, excluding depreciation and interest
Accounts payable	30 days of nonsalary expenses, excluding depreciation and interest
Accrued liabilities	15 days of salary expenses

Analytical Steps

The reader should now perform the following analysis:

- Determine annual cash flows.

- Develop potential assumptions related to the alternative financing methods.

- Discount cash flows at a rate based on the material presented in this chapter.

- Evaluate the construction project and determine the appropriate financing method.

Chapter 12

Current Environmental Issues

INTRODUCTION

Environmental pressures have a direct impact on the financial organization and operations of a hospital. It is difficult to cite the most important pressures. However, three issues are receiving increasing attention in the hospital field and promise to have continuing, long-range impacts on the financial environment in which hospitals function: the annual hospital report (AHR), IRS audits and reporting requirements, and risk management related to malpractice and self-insurance.

At this writing, the AHR may not become a complete reality. Congress, under pressure from the health care industry and influenced by cost studies that reported significant costs associated with the system, has denied HHS funding for the project. However, there are significant issues in the proposal that should be understood by hospital administrations: functional rather than responsibility reporting, uniform recording of data, direct allocation of overhead, and direct matching of statistics with accounting data. These are matters that hospitals should be aware of when threatened by governmental regulation. They also should be understood by hospitals in terms of their potential internal use as enhancements to current management systems.

With respect to IRS relations and reporting, in 1977, not-for-profit hospitals were required to submit Form 990 (Return of Organizations Exempt from Income Tax). This focused the hospital industry's attention on continued compliance with IRS regulations and on a reexamination of the internal operations of hospitals that might be in questionable compliance with regulations. The IRS began an intensive investigation of key areas of compliance. With this background, it is extremely important that hospitals investigate and weigh heavily the tax aspects of decisions and operations in the administrative process.

The dramatic increase in medical malpractice insurance premiums has caused the industry to seek alternative forms of insurance coverage. Among these alternatives are risk-management programs and self-insurance trusts based on actuarial studies of individual loss experience. Risk-management programs require direct administrative involvement in the establishment and evaluation of sound policies and procedures related to patient care and the maintenance of safe environmental conditions.

IRS REPORTING AND RELATIONS

The basic tax reporting requirement for the not-for-profit institution is the use of the Form 990 (Return of Organizations Exempt from Income Tax). The emphasis of this return is on the operations of the institution in accordance with applicable tax guidelines in the law and IRS regulations.

The IRS has indicated that hospitals will be targeted for intensive compliance review in future years. Church hospitals are particularly vulnerable, since they began to file returns for the first time in 1976. The IRS is looking for situations where a hospital's directors, officers, trustees, or employees are engaging in transactions that could be characterized as "self-dealing." It is paying particular attention to physician compensation arrangements and to unrelated business income, for example, income from doctor's offices, parking lots used by the general public, cafeterias and coffee shops selling to the general public, cooperative hospital service organizations, and pharmacy sales.

Generally, the IRS agent first looks to see whether or not the hospital is a "public-charity" type of organization, that is, whether it is rendering services to the general public. The agent then looks at the books and records to find out whether there have been any dealings between the hospital and closely related persons. The agent will look at contributions to the hospital and at deductions taken by persons outside the hospital and will examine employee records and hospital-based physician arrangements that might involve tax withholdings that have not been reported for the individuals by the hospital. All operations of the hospital will be reviewed for unrelated business income and for compliance with Revenue Ruling 69–545, including admitting and treatment practices in the emergency room.

The hospital must therefore maintain adequate and complete records related to all financial operations of the institution. Care must be taken to establish clear policies that identify all operational aspects of the institution that are in compliance with IRS regulations.

RISK MANAGEMENT

In the past, institutions that sought protection against medical malpractice and public liability losses transferred the risks to commercial insurance underwriters at economically acceptable premiums with modest deductibles. Now, however, because of the trend toward "social inflation"—extending liability to areas where it did not exist before and establishing new standards for putting values on traditional liabilities—losses, especially in the field of medical malpractice, have become unpredictably large, and premiums have responded accordingly. The result is that the premiums, if attainable or quotable at all, are no longer economically advantageous. Therefore, alternatives must be considered. These include total self-insurance or self-insurance with excess insurance coverage to stop the per-occurrence loss at some predetermined level.

Considering the present excess premium now being charged, the expectation of substantial renewal premium increases, and the good loss experience, total self-insurance is a viable alternative to the present medical malpractice and public liability program in terms of reducing the overall costs and allowing cash flow advantages. For example, suppose a hospital's year-loss experience has been $192,000 for medical malpractice and public liability. These figures include paid losses and reserves. The cash flow advantages may be evidenced by the fact that only $76,980 has been paid over the past three years for medical malpractice and public liability claims.

Risk-management programs have been designed around the pending revised rules in the Provider Reimbursement Manual (HIM–15), Part I, so that administrative fees may be reimbursable. In short, the rules state that Medicare will permit reimbursement for contributions to a trusteed self-insurance reserve fund established by a provider that self-insures to protect itself against the risk of medical malpractice and to obtain reimbursement of its related administrative costs. At this writing, the relevant provision is scheduled to be altered to allow only for contributions based on actual Medicare claims on an historic basis, not in total as before.

A risk-management system includes risk-management administration, claims management, claims evaluation and accounting, claims investigation, actuarial services and evaluation, financial management, insurance placement, loss control/safety training, and coordination of legal requirements.

Because of the number of persons required to provide the specialized services in a risk-management system, it is necessary that one person be responsible for coordinating all the various related activities. Usually, a risk-management administrator is assigned this responsibility to obtain the best delivery in the flow of services and to achieve the optimum performance. The key to effective performance of self-insurance administration is communications; and, to a great degree, the key to effective communications is understanding. That is, the people involved must understand the objectives, their own roles, and how they relate within the overall program. At inception, the objectives—overall and specific—should be established for each operating group.

The service structure of claims investigation, claims evaluation, safety and loss control, statistical and actuarial services, financial management, and legal representatives could become cumbersome if it is not tightly coordinated by the risk management administrator. Therefore, regularly scheduled meetings between the external consultant, hospital representatives, and the risk management administrator are imperative. Just how frequently these meetings should be held may be difficult to determine. Initially, regularly scheduled biweekly internal meetings should be held with the external consultants group, and biweekly or, at the very least, monthly meetings should be held between the hospital's designated representatives and the external administrator. The subject matter and format of these meetings should not become so formal that they become mechanical. However, each meeting should include reports from each service manager concerning the following segments of the program:

- the overall status of the area of responsibility

- the action that the consultant will be able to take to respond to the hospital's stated goal

- the status of any hospital input data or action on which the consultant's future activities are dependent

- the nature of any new developments and plans to respond to them

- general descriptions of new approaches, techniques, or services that could enhance the hospital's program

- discussion of any areas of concern that could become future trouble areas or require a new response from the hospital.

Obviously, the day-to-day routine work will be done within the consultant's various operating groups and departments by personnel who should be in direct contact with representatives of the hospital. It should be the responsibility of each service manager to see that this work is performed efficiently and professionally. This should become a part of the managers' regular reports to management on the overall status of their areas of responsibility. It should be the responsibility of the risk management administrator to coordinate all relevant activities and to make certain that the full scope of expertise, services, and attention is brought to bear on a timely basis. This will make the self-insurance program a truly effective program that is constantly improving its benefits to the hospital.

Procedures for accomplishing for a health care facility an evaluation of the administrative aspects of medical malpractice commence with interviews with administrative staff, department heads, health care and other line personnel, on down to relatively new employees. The principal objective is to measure the hospital against its own standards, as established in corporation bylaws, medical staff bylaws, departmental policies and procedures, and so on. The emphasis should be on knowledge of procedures, orientation and training of employees, controls, incident reporting and analysis, and, above all, administrative interest and direction. Through the evaluation, recommendations of an administrative nature are developed which, when implemented, will serve to enhance the defense posture of the hospital with regard to the medical malpractice claims. The evaluation is directed at administrative functions; normally it is not related to the medical aspects of malpractice.

Hospitals are deeply concerned with the safety and well-being of their patients, visitors, students, and employees and the protection of their fixed assets. The following services are required in connection with these concerns:

- evaluation of the administrative aspects of medical malpractice control

- assistance to the hospital administration in the development of viable and comprehensive safety programs with the objective of meeting new standards of the Joint Commission for the Accreditation of Hospitals (JCAH)

- evaluation of physical plants regarding general liability exposures and controls with special emphasis addressed to the Life Safety Code.

The administration of the hospital should consider the adoption of a "total loss control program" encompassing all elements of potential injury or damage. Consultants have found that segmenting loss control responsibilities is a deterrent to sound safety management. From an administrative standpoint, it is inappropriate to assign to separate management units those elements of loss control that should be included as a part of total loss control, malpractice control, fire safety and control, emergency planning, disaster planning, and security. The fact that many incidents cut across several loss control areas supports this argument. For example, a fall is the most prevalent type of incident in studies of employee, patient, student, and visitor loss experience. If a worker's compensation claim and a medical malpractice claim arise out of the same patient-handling incident, the object for management treatment is patient handling, not employee safety or medical malpractice. If a diathermy machine has an electrical short that goes unattended and a nurse, patient, or student is shocked, the subject is electrical equipment maintenance. A fire presents risk of injury to patients, visitors, students, and employees and very often also affects security. Furthermore:

- Management concepts necessary to achieve good programs are the same, whatever the injury or damage potential.

- Disciplines involved in achieving a good level of loss control in each field are related.

- All control programs are accomplished through the same management people.

Given most organizational structures, administrative people are required to treat individual safety subjects separately rather than as a part of a coordinated program. When several people are assigned responsibility for individual segments of the loss control effort, performance levels vary greatly. Communications among those responsible for the control of injury or damage potential present a most serious problem that will not be resolved unless there is a single direction of loss control activity and a single organization that brings involved people together for discussion and resolution of all safety and loss control subjects.

Claims management covers the critical areas of claims reporting, investigating, evaluation, and settlement. Usually, the external consultant will receive, record, and analyze all claims or potential claims in the hospital's behalf. In this role, the consultant should review all incident reports on a regular basis to determine the claim potential and, when necessary, assign the claim to a professional claims investigation and adjustment service. All such assignments should be confirmed in writing to the hospital. All investigations should be coordinated through the hospital's designated representative. Following the claims assignment, the consultant should receive and review all investigation reports and evaluate the facts, recommendations, and reserves suggested by the external adjustment service. Upon review, the consultant should establish a recommended claim reserve and make necessary recommendations relative to settlement.

It is generally recommended that the hospital establish an in-house claim committee consisting of professional, administrative, financial, and legal personnel. This unit can recommend and assist in the selection of an attorney for legal advice and in the necessary defense of litigated claims. The claims evaluation unit should utilize the reports from the consultant's statistical unit as the basis for an ongoing program to identify, analyze, and evaluate the exposures, losses, causes, and methods of reducing or controlling the risks of the hospital, in conjunction with the external consultants.

The soaring cost of medical malpractice liability insurance, coupled with the shrinking capacity and withdrawal of the commercial insurance markets, has created the need for a major reappraisal by many medical institutions of available funding alternatives.

Under a self-insurance program, a fund should be established to pay for anticipated losses. Actuarial studies are used to determine the proper amount of money required by this fund. The prime requisite of the consultant's study should be to establish the proper level of expected losses for the institution. This determination is made in three steps:

- A risk-analysis survey of the historical loss experience of hospitals is performed.

- The data compiled by a national statistical and rate-making organization, is usually reviewed to determine the loss expectancy on a class-average basis. Projections based on frequency and severity levels and trends are made.

- The experience of the hospital is compared to the class-average base to determine the expected variation.

In addition, a cash flow analysis of the recommended funding approach should be made in order to demonstrate the capacity of the program in handling adverse variations in actual results. Finally, the consultant should present the conclusions of the study, including the background and concepts involved.

The statistical reporting unit should work in conjunction with the claims management unit to provide detailed statistical analyses of claims incidents. These reports should provide a means of continuously monitoring the factors giving rise to the incidents and the data concerning the stage and timing of claims payment processing. In this connection, the consultant should provide continuous monitoring of disbursement procedures and a profile of all claims to facilitate accurate reserve judgments. In addition, the statistical analyses should provide a sound base for the development of programs to lessen the incidence of malpractice claims. Finally, the statistical reporting unit should work with the financial management unit to create an informative environment for the varied funding aspects of the program. This process should enhance the creation of the least costly and most fully covered risk management situation for the hospital.

In the broadest sense, financial management of the hospital self-insurance trust fund should cover all financial operations of the fund, policy-setting as well as implementation. In this context, in seeking to support the credibility of an arms-length relationship between the hospital and the fund administration, the consultant should be qualified to serve as the financial policy maker of the fund, representing the interests of the hospital in establishing the trust, developing its goals and objectives, and carrying out its day-to-day financial operations and obligations. At the same time, the consultant should maintain a constant awareness and control of both revenue and costs so that the interests of the hospital, as well as the interests of ultimate claimants, are best served.

The trust administrator usually reserves the right to recommend and (in harmony with the hospital) select and/or replace trustees working in the context of the trust agreements. In conjunction with the overall plan administration, the trustees should be willing to work with the consultants in assuming responsibilities in the following basic areas of trust financial management:

- collection

- accounting

- auditing

- financial reporting

- investment performance review

- state and federal reporting compliance

In the context of sound trust financial management, the consultant should:

- administer the trust

- guide the protection of the trust property

- facilitate the payment of approved claim settlements

- review the productivity of trust property

- expedite collection of funds due the trust

- account for the handling of all trust funds

The prudent management of trust monies is a vital element of fiduciary responsibility providing many interesting challenges to both trustees and administrators.

The risk management program should provide for continued insurance placement review. Through continual involvement in the market place, the hospital is assured of continued financial advantages in maintaining the risk management program and the self-insurance posture.

REORGANIZATION ISSUES

Current economic problems in the United States touch every aspect of people's lives. The effects are felt in constantly changing government regulations and budget cuts as well as in everincreasing prices for food and clothing. The problems also affect the business world, where executives attempt to continue production and services while faced with spiraling interest rates and supply costs. The hospital industry has not been immune to these societal and economic forces.

In the past, hospitals were described as a cottage industry. Usually, each hospital was a separate corporation, providing services to the public as it decided. For many such institutions, it was a time of growth in physical plant, new technological equipment, and innovative programs. Each hospital was governed by a single, self-perpetuating board that delegated the administrative and medical care responsibilities to a single management and single medical staff respectively. As previously discussed, a large proportion of the hospitals were organized as not-for-profit, tax-exempt corporations under Section 501(c)(3) of the Internal Revenue Service Tax Code. In addition to their revenues, they depended on charitable contributions and, in more recent years, on tax-exempt bond financing as necessary sources of cash.

But the changes in the hospital's external environment have been many and diverse. The federal government has become an ever larger third party reimburser of health care. Thus, the hospital's financial viability is very dependent on the actions of the government, especially when budget cutting or decreased dollars for health care are proposed.

In addition, new health planning laws now require certificate-of-need approval for capital expansion. In many states, hospitals now face rate regulation by a state agency, which further serves to inhibit the free operation of the hospital as a private corporation. Finally, the IRS has increased its surveillance of hospitals, especially in the area of unrelated business income and subsequent loss of tax-exempt status. All of these factors, combined with increasing competition, litigation, and rising interest rates, are forcing many hospital executives to look for innovative ways to survive in the modern environment.

One organizational strategy proposed as a solution is corporate reorganization. Such reorganization allows hospitals "to abandon outdated organizational structures and create broad, multi-corporation social institutions that will allow them to maximize hospital reimbursement, protect their assets and expand services without government interference."[1] However, like any major program, reorganization requires a great deal of preliminary work.

One of the most important elements in restructuring is planning. "A hospital has to have a good long-range plan for services and capital development to know what form its corporate organization should take."[2] The consideration of corporate reorganization by a hospital's management means changes in the basic philosophy underlying the mission of a health care institution. It means that all involved must have definite plans and goals for the hospital and for its continued survival. The planning stage must also address how the community will react to such changes and how to be prepared to meet with opposition.

An integral part of such planning is the financial aspect of reorganization. Often, the hospital has come to the need for reorganization because of decreasing cash flow. Many hospitals are having covenant clauses written into their tax-exempt bonds to allow for the transfer of assets.[3] This gives the hospital the freedom to reorganize later without having to refinance the bond issue at higher interest rates. With this barrier removed, the hospital can begin to separate out nonpatient care areas or ancillary activity areas that adversely affect reimbursement. Frequently, these separated activities can then be conducted as revenue-producing activities that might gain from the new form of organization.[4] Here, financial considerations must include the question of tax status for the new corporation. It may be decided that one or more areas should not be tax-exempt but taxable and profit-making.

As noted earlier, the community response to proposed reorganization plans must be elicited and monitored. The community response can begin with those community representatives on the governing board and/or the advisory board, but it must ultimately involve a more representative sample of the community served. One group that will be affected are the other providers in the area, since reorganization can alter previously established relationships.[5]

Another important question to answer is, "Who should be involved?" While the impetus for reorganization usually comes from the administration or the board, a much broader range of players needs to be involved at some time during the process. The "process must be accomplished in conjunction with those most affected by any restructuring, including the hospital's community, administration, medical staff, and employees; and with other health services providers, planners, financial and reimbursement specialists. . . ."[6] An additional participant is the corporate law attorney, who knows what is and is not regulated by federal or state statutes. Each of these persons and groups will supply different kinds of input at various stages of the reorganization. Clearly the health care institution does not exist as a lone corporation in a vast wilderness but as an entity in a complex environment with innumerable relationships.

The restructuring process has three basic parts: (1) the preliminary steps, (2) the corporate study, and (3) the development of proposals. The preliminary steps include educating the board with a broad interdisciplinary approach, especially if the proposal did not originate with the board; assembling a team of advisors; and finally forming a steering committee to act in both consultative and administrative capacities during the early stages. The corporate study phase will necessitate the development of a list of key objectives and an analysis of the existing corporate structure. The final phase concerns the various proposals that must be developed. This will begin with interviewing and regulatory research and analysis, followed by a financial analysis. The preliminary proposals are then developed, and the draft study is completed. The last step involves the presentation and discussion of the final report. Upon acceptance of this final report, the reorganization becomes a reality.

The new corporate organization will usually be representative of one of three basic types of institution: independent foundations, parent holding company, or multiple entities. Often these types are used in combinations that will best serve the needs of the hospital. Each type has its own major purpose and benefit/cost trade-offs.

The first is the independent foundation, illustrated in Figure 12-1 as an entity separate from the hospital. Both the hospital and the foundation are usually tax-exempt organizations under Section 501(c)(3). The independent foundation is often used for fund raising or business ventures. It also ensures the hospital that its endowment assets are properly sheltered. It achieves its maximum utility when used as a safeguard from the regulatory process. Its biggest disadvantage is the hospital's loss of control over the foundation's activities.

The second type is the parent holding company. As illustrated in Figure 12-2, this type is patterned after the bankholding corporation, in which case assets belong to the parent, not to a single member hospital. Again, in this design both entities are tax-exempt under Section 501(c)(3). Usually the parent company not only controls the assets but the board is transferred from the member to the parent. The hospital deals only with patient care items, and its financial reporting consists of the statement of revenue and expenses for such items. In addition to the total assets of the corporation, the parent has both the nonpatient care areas and the largely nonreimbursable areas. This type organization allows for a separation of activities, while retaining control over the total operations. In this context, joint financial reporting is possible.

Figure 12–1 The Independent Foundation

Figure 12–2 The Parent Holding Company

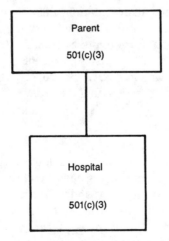

The third type of corporate organization, multiple entities, provides the widest variety of structures with the best chance of adaptation to a specific case. The entities often go through at least one interim phase before achieving the "right" organization. One possible resultant structure is shown in Figure 12–3. In this case, the strategy was to separate those areas that might suffer from being together with the hospital. Sales and services is an area that sells to its own employees. As a separate entity, the revenue collected there is not unrelated business income, although the corporation can still maintain its Section 501(c)(3) eligibility. The parent can accumulate the excess revenue and distribute it to the hospital, without affecting either its own tax status or the tax status of the hospital.

An example of a sophisticated reorganization is that of multiple entities with mixed tax statuses. This might involve a hospital that has a good endowment program, an excess capacity of top management ability and a psychiatric clinic and is looking for acquisitions. The resulting structure may appear as in Figure 12–4.

Figure 12–3 The Multiple-Entity Corporation

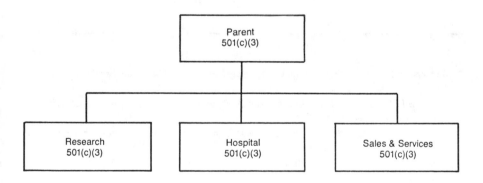

Figure 12-4 The Multiple-Entity Corporation—Mixed Tax Status

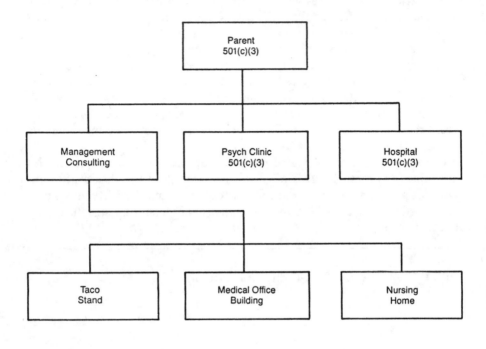

NOTES

1. Suzanne LaViolette, "Snowed under by Regs, Hospitals Unbundle Services," *Modern Healthcare* 10: 52.
2. Suzanne LaViolette, "Eager Hospitals Tackle Politics, Emotions Raised by Restructuring Plans," *Modern Healthcare* 10: 58.
3. Donna Leith Yanish, "Hospital Bond Issue Design Ensures Corporate Restructuring Freedom," *Modern Healthcare* 10: 62.
4. David H. Hill and Michael P. Harrishthal, "Financing Health Care in the 1980's," *Hospitals, JAHA* 54: 74.
5. John N. Halfield II, "Restructuring: A Responsible Alternative to Hospital Closure," *Trustee* 33: 34.
6. Ibid.

Part IV

Financial Planning

The key to a hospital's financial success in the current environment is financial planning, as evidenced by the current emphasis on prospective rate reviews. Today's hospital must have an integrated, systematic framework for the development of a financial plan that is flexible enough to change with environmental developments. There are a variety of techniques, time frames, and philosophies applicable to the hospital financial planning process. These include statistical techniques, such as time-series, exponential smoothing, and regression analysis, that are used in a variety of financial models and forecast types. Time frames vary from the short range of less than one year to the long range spanning several years. Financial plans may range from fixed to flexible and from department responsibility to program budget. Our purpose in this section is to provide an overview of the financial planning environment, including an analysis of various techniques and approaches in common use.

Chapter 13 provides an overview of the budgeting process. The various philosophies of fixed, flexible, responsibility, and zero-based budgeting are discussed. Approaches to a financial planning system are illustrated in the case of the budgeting system of Community Medical Center.

Chapter 14 is devoted to forecasting statistics that form the basis for a large part of the financial planning process. Techniques include time-series decomposition, exponential smoothing, and regression analysis. The use of each technique is illustrated in the case study.

Chapter 15 discusses cost analysis and projections to be formulated into a systematic mode of rate of return identification and rate setting. An analysis of costs relates activity to cost on an inflation-adjusted historic basis, utilizing "high/low" and regression analysis techniques. This analysis simplifies the budgeting and control process and forms the basis for flexible budgeting.

Various types of cost behavior—fixed, variable, and semivariable—are described. In this context, break-even points and the general financial requirements of hospitals are examined, as outlined by the American Hospital Association. An analysis of project rate setting is developed in a discussion of internal rate-of-return requirements.

Chapter 16 concentrates on the development and use of pro forma financial statements and the increasing use of financial forecasting models. Financial interrelationships and pro forma financial statements are discussed and illustrated in the case of Community Medical Center.

Chapter 13

Budgeting and Financial Planning Concepts

INTRODUCTION

Financial planning provides the framework for guiding managerial decisions and evaluating operating results. Financial planning takes various forms and degrees of formality over a wide range of time frames. The form of a financial plan may be categorized by operational flexibility—for example, a fixed or flexible budget—or by control unit—for example, departmental responsibility or program budget. There are also varying degrees of personnel and physician involvement in the budgeting process. Finally, in the emerging concept of zero-based budgeting, each area is evaluated and reevaluated as to purpose and benefits relative to costs and organizational goals and objectives. Our purpose here is to introduce various approaches to financial planning and to evaluate each approach based on the managerial advantages and disadvantages inherent in a particular system or philosophy.

COMPONENTS OF FINANCIAL PLANNING

The components of a financial plan are operationally oriented in that the basic framework for a planning system relates to the logical flows of financial data. While revenues and expenses are key elements of operational performance, increasing emphasis is being placed on cash flow and cash planning, which represent the culmination of overall operational effectiveness.

It is managerially important that the planning format be designed to address key elements that are useful in monitoring financial operating results on either a program or responsibility basis. While activity projections are essential to the establishment of staffing patterns and expense, revenue, and capital projections, it may be argued that staffing and expenses are the key elements of control. Efficient staffing patterns and justification criteria, combined with industrial engineering studies that are required before new positions are approved and even before vacancies are filled, are the most controllable elements of financial operations. To be useful in a control function, a financial plan must identify controllable and uncontrollable elements of revenues and expenses.

From a management viewpoint, it is essential that those persons having responsibility for expenditures and daily operations be directly involved in the planning process. This involvement is not limited to departmental managers and administration. It should also include the medical staff and community leaders who, in one sense, are the hospital's market and, in another sense, are closely tied to community needs. Continuous communication is required between the administration and responsible middle managers, not only during initial planning but throughout the budget year so that any variances or changes in environmental conditions may be evaluated and action taken to minimize any disruptive effects on fiscal viability.

FIXED VERSUS FLEXIBLE BUDGETS

Usually, a hospital projects a particular level of patient activity—for example, patient days and ancillary visits or procedures—and projects all revenues, expenses, and deductions based on this one level of activity. Such an approach is used in the preparation of a "fixed" budget. As hospitals have become increasingly aware that activity is not directly controllable within a particular responsibility area, a variation on the fixed budget has evolved. This approach recognizes the fact that expenses increase and decrease with changes and fluctuations in departmental activity. Furthermore, not all expenses vary directly with changes in activity. Consequently, in this approach, expenses are classified by activity correlation. Those expenses that vary directly with activity are categorized as variable, those that do not vary with activity are classified as fixed, and those that vary in step increments over activity ranges are identified as semivariable, which is synonymous with semifixed.

The fixed budget is the easiest to project, given the extreme complexity of the hospital operation. Each department provides a multitude of services that operate and interact within an overall patient care environment. Consequently, it is difficult at best to identify and classify specific, incremental costs. To a significant degree, hospitals provide services on at least a standby level, which results in a significant proportion of total costs being fixed over a relevant range of activity.

Conversely, a fixed budget is set at one particular activity level. There is no allowance made for expense fluctuations due to activity. It is possible that, under a fixed budget, a department will have no variance in budgeted expenditures. This may not be a readily identifiable problem, even though activity for the area has been reduced substantially. Whether or not this is a problem requiring managerial intervention may be difficult to determine, since it is not known how expenditures are expected to fluctuate with activity.

An increasing number of hospitals are exploring flexible budgets. In this connection, it should be remembered that a sound and valid fixed budget is managerially more valuable that a "poor" flexible budget. However, hospitals should be aware of the potential of flexible budgeting as a powerful planning and control tool, given the validity of cost analysis on a sound and reasonable basis.

PROGRAM VERSUS RESPONSIBILITY BUDGETS

As we have seen, the typical hospital is organized functionally, with each specific function identified as a cost center or department. Examples are radiology, housekeeping, business office, and maintenance. Generally, each department is viewed as a distinct organizational unit with its own budget and statements related to that department's operations. Usually, the department manager is responsible for adhering to the budget for the area for which the manager is responsible. Such an approach to budget preparation and subsequent performance monitoring is referred to as responsibility budgeting.

It will be remembered that in the case of project cash flows and program evaluation, each program is segmented as a separate functional project containing revenues from project operations and total expenses in all areas serving the program. Logically, a medical patient occupies a bed requiring not only routine nursing and support services but also ancillary services such as radiology, laboratory, pharmacy, and respiratory therapy. A further development of this approach identifies services required by diagnosis. Here the basis for budgeting is the projection of diagnoses and therefore of related services of ancillaries and support areas. The budget then becomes one, not for a segmentized area, but for a patient-oriented program for care by diagnosis or service project. This approach to budget organization is known as program budgeting.

The responsibility budget has managerial benefits in that a single person is responsible for adhering to a unique financial plan. Control directly interfaces with the typical organization structure. The responsibility budget has a further advantage in that financial reporting is usually maintained on a departmental basis, which provides direct budget-versus-actual comparisons. Costs by department are easily accumulated, given the centralized nature of staffing and expense incurrence on a departmental basis. However, the responsibility budget does not reflect the interrelated nature of the services provided in its principle product, patient care.

The program budget is segmented by hospital service function. This segmentation is based on treatment of patients and ties directly into the product orientation of the hospital—treatment of specific patient categories of need. Revenues and costs identified by service area provide a direct insight into the hospital's program costs. Such information is managerially useful in that a standard is developed by treatment modality, through diagnoses that provide identification of cost. Such cost may be directly related to revenue to provide for an equitable charge structure and for identification via the financial system of extraordinary treatment modalities for managerial investigation.

While sound in theory, the program budget has found little widespread use in hospitals, due primarily to the vast array of services that are interrelated with various diagnoses and alternative treatment programs. There is significant difficulty in cost allocation from a responsibility-accumulation basis to a program basis. Staffing is not based on the incremental base of diagnoses, nor is expense incurrence recorded in terms of this categorization. Expenses are incurred on a departmental basis, even though they are directly associated with overall patient care and diagnosis treatments.

In summary, the responsibility budget will probably continue to be the most widely used budget system in the near future. However, activity projections based on general treatment statistics provide a sound step toward program budgeting. For example, psychiatric patients as a general rule utilize fewer ancillary services per patient day than do medical/surgical patients. Recognition of this in projecting ancillary activity, which may be based on total patient days or admissions, is an easily utilized aspect of program budgeting.

ZERO-BASED BUDGETING

Zero-based budgeting has been described as a revolutionary management tool in budget system design. However, some critics view this concept as a fad, as merely a synonym for sound managerial practices, that will soon fade away. In any event, zero-based budgeting does not solve all managerial problems, and it cannot be used effectively unless the system is properly designed and patterned to interface with an organizational decision-making need.

Zero-based budgeting consists of four basic phases. The first phase subdivides the organization into groups of discrete units. These units may be departments, cost centers, or subdivisions, depending on the organization of the institution. The second phase is the analysis of each of the segments to determine what the objectives of the segment are and the current and alternative procedures for achieving those objectives. Once the best method of operation has been determined, the analysis identifies several activity levels at which the unit could function. This process starts with a base level, which is usually below current activity; and levels are added incrementally, usually until activities are above current volumes. For each level added, the analysis identifies costs and benefits associated with the addition of the level.

In the third phase, managers rank the incremental levels and develop an overall set of organizational priorities. At this point, dollars are associated with the service phases, and a ceiling is placed on overall expenditures. Those levels ranked highest are accepted; those that are ranked below funding levels are rejected. Once this process is completed, in the fourth phase, the operating budgets are prepared for each decision unit, and the results are communicated to the appropriate management personnel.

There are several reasons why an organization may find it advantageous to utilize zero-based budgeting. First, each area is analyzed to a finite degree as to basic services and the alternatives for providing those services. Managers are forced through this process to review completely the operations of their areas and to communicate their analysis to administrative personnel. There is an advantage to such an analysis, in that nonproductive services and operational practices are identified and a decision can be made as to continuing the operation or utilizing the funds for a higher ranking level of activity, possibly even in another area of the institution.

The most critical time in the development of a zero-based budget system is the time of implementation. The conversion process should be systematic, and managers should be trained in procedures to achieve the most significant impact from the program.

Critics argue that it is almost impossible to utilize fully the zero-based concept in areas of management and in the direct, general care of the patient. For example, it is easy to develop levels of activity in such areas of production as housekeeping, where the base level of activity may be the minimum cleaning level of the patient care areas and subsequent levels can be based on the number of times the areas are cleaned and when to clean nonpatient areas. However, in nursing the base level of care is almost impossible to identify. If incremental benefits to patient care were available, the hospital would as a matter of operational practice acquire the process.

Still, the hospital should keep in mind the basic concept behind zero-based budgeting, that is, sound managerial communication and continuous evaluation of operations in a cost-effective manner.

LONG-RANGE PLANNING

Each hospital should have a formalized long-range financial plan to monitor current progress and to quantify overall trends in the organization and in the area served. The long-range plan may take a variety of forms. However, the most useful plans begin with an identification of the goals and objectives of the organization and a matching of these goals with the demographics of the area served. All alternatives should be explored, and all personnel associated with the hospital should be involved in the identification of future trends in treatment and in activity and service levels.

The quantification of these trends should reflect current operations and be based on a simple model of individual department operations. Gross pro forma financial statements are useful in the identification of key relationships in the financial statements and operations and can provide an indication of the overall trends in future financial operations.

PLANNING COMPONENTS

A sound financial plan includes the following components:

- activity projections
- expense projections
- capital expenditures projections
- revenue and cash flow projections

Each of these components must be developed in an organized system for the collection of historic data and the development of projections for services offered and activities to be experienced over the planning horizon.

In the development of the system, all persons connected with the hospital must be actively involved. It is absolutely necessary to have direct involvement in the budget development by those managers who will be held accountable for future performance. The most significant group in influencing hospital activity and services is the medical staff. All physicians should be asked to provide input into the process, with responsibility as available for monitoring future performance.

COMMUNITY MEDICAL CENTER: FINANCIAL PLANNING

Figure 13–1 shows the budget flows for Community Medical Center. Note the involvement of all areas of the institution. The process involves a fixed budget predicated on certain facts and assumptions:

- an average daily census of 322, totaling 117,530 patient days, compared with an average daily census of 316 or 115,340 patient days in 1976

- an average growth rate of 5 percent in ancillary services

- increases in F.I.C.A. limits, Blue Cross coverage, unemployment compensation, and insurance fees averaging approximately 16 percent

- contractual allowances totaling 50 percent of adjusted net income, and bad debt reserves at 5 percent of gross charges

- a 7 percent salary increase effective January 1977

- inclusion of employee life insurance coverage

- an average inflation rate of 9 percent in supplies

- a prorated increase in man hours and mix of personnel based on new and improved services

- capital expenditures that reflect replacements and new services, such as an upgraded laboratory, along with future construction requirements

- an average rate increase of approximately 9 percent

Present legislation, for example P.L. 92–603 and P.L. 93–641 affects current operations and planning, and JCAH requirements place a financial stress on health care institutions. As a result, the center is anticipating an increase in the general care room rate of $5.00/day or 6.7 percent and 8.5 percent (average) in ancillary areas. These increases are lower than in previous budgets and may have to be changed to conform with regulations, such as Medicare's "lower of costs or charges" rulings.

However, the center continues to maintain flexibility within an ever-changing structure in line with financial objectives established by the governing board. Monthly monitoring of budget-versus-actual experience continues to be the center's practice in maintaining a healthy financial position.

The center's budget, based on the above data, is to be presented to the center's board. It is the reader's responsibility as president of the center to make the presentation for 1980. The reader should be prepared to defend not only the facts contained in the budget but the philosophies used in the projections. In the preparation of points to be used in the presentation, the following questions should be addressed: What areas should be presented in the meeting? What approach should be taken in preparing the budget?

The reader should prepare a summary analysis of the budget, utilizing previous data on the historic operations of the center. The feasibility summary for the center in Chapter 11 should serve as a reference point in the analysis. Finally, the reader should develop summary results of the budget preparation, for example, a statement of revenues and expenses.

Figure 13–1 Budget Flows for Community Medical Center

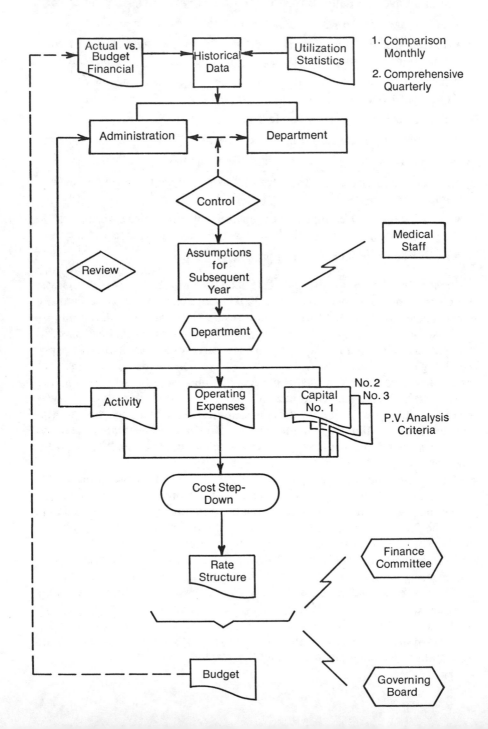

Chapter 14

Forecasting Statistics

INTRODUCTION

As we have noted, the basis for a financial plan is the statistics related to the activity of the various areas of the institution. It is essential that both revenues and expenses be based on statistics that relate directly to the financial data to be forecasted. Techniques in common use in forecasting statistics range from a "best guess" method, which draws on general impressions of persons familiar with the operations of the area to be forecasted, to advanced statistical techniques, including time-series decomposition, exponential smoothing, and regression analysis.

Apart from these statistical techniques, one should not discount the importance of the subjective element in forecasting. Often, forecasting activity is based on a subjective estimation derived from a detailed knowledge of the institution on the part of those responsible for projections and operations. Many of the criticisms of fully quantitative techniques are best handled by judgments as to the reasonableness of the quantitative forecast.

The following discussion of two of the three quantitative techniques for forecasting statistics mentioned above—time-series decomposition and regression analysis—is presented at a relatively simple level, with more advanced applications left to further research by the reader.

TIME-SERIES DECOMPOSITION

Decomposition methods use the history of a particular series of data to forecast future values in the series. For example, the hospital may want to use historical patient days to predict patient days for the next quarter, or it may want to use the seasonal pattern of deliveries for previous years to predict the seasonal pattern for the coming year.

A time series can be viewed as a collection of trend, seasonal, and irregular components. Decomposition analysis involves the estimation of the various components and the preparation of forecasts based on these estimates.

Decomposition is the easiest of time-series techniques when a single forecast is required. Other techniques, such as exponential smoothing, are more economical when repeated forecasts are required.

However, decomposition techniques fail to consider casual relationships with outside factors that may affect the dependent variable being forecasted. The basic assumption underlying decomposition is that past patterns and causal factors will continue to operate in the future. Therefore, it is impossible to predict turning points other than seasonal variations, and this limits the use of the technique to short-term forecasts, usually three months or less.

REGRESSION ANALYSIS

The simple linear equation $Y_t = A + BX_t + u_t$ states that in period t the value of Y, the dependent variable, is determined by four factors: the population constant A; the population regression coefficient B; the level of X, which is the independent variable; and the level u, which is the sum of all the other factors that influence Y, each of which is assumed to be of minor importance. The equation is simple because only one independent variable is used to compute the dependent variable and because it is linear. Note that Y is defined by only the one independent variable X that bears some linear relationship to Y.

Simple least-squares regression analysis is a technique for estimating A and B from a set of sample values of X and Y. The least-squares technique yields estimates with the property that, for a sample, the sum of the squares of the residuals is minimized. A residual is the difference between an actual and a fitted value of the dependent variable, where the fitted value for the period t is given by $(a + bX_t)$.

Simple regression analysis has great flexibility in application. For example, it can be used to estimate a linear trend by defining X as time, measured from a value of 1 in the first period, which corresponds to the first observed value of X to a value of n in the final or nth period. It should be noted that a linear trend can also be estimated by other means. One method is to draw a line through a set of plotted points of the dependent variable versus the independent variable. Another method is to compute the average of the first few values of the dependent variable and the average of the last few values and then fit the trend through these averages. The reason for calculating the trend by the least-squares regression is that the trend fitted in this way has the property that the sum of the squares of the deviations for the entire period is minimized.

The values for a and b are computed by application of the following formulas to the set of data under analysis:

$$b = \frac{\sum\limits_{t=1}^{n} X_t Y_t - \left(\left(\sum\limits_{t=1}^{n} X_t \right) \left(\sum\limits_{t=1}^{n} Y_t \right) / n \right)}{\sum\limits_{t=1}^{n} X_t^2 - \left(\left(\sum\limits_{t=1}^{n} X_t \right)^2 / n \right)}$$

$$a = \bar{Y} - b\bar{X} = \left(\left(\sum\limits_{t=1}^{n} Y_t \right) / n \right) - b \left(\left(\sum\limits_{t=1}^{n} X_t \right) / n \right)$$

The correlation coefficient R and the square of that measure R^2 are summary statistics of the "goodness of fit" or explanatory power of the estimated equation. They are computed from sample data. Specifically, R^2 shows the proportion of the variance of Y in the sample that is accounted for by the estimating equation:

$$R^2 = \left(\sum\limits_{t=1}^{n} (\hat{Y}_t - \bar{Y})^2 / \sum\limits_{t=1}^{n} (Y_t - \bar{Y})^2 \right)$$

Here, the numerator is the sum of the squares of the deviations of the fitted values of Y_t ($\hat{Y}_t$) from the sample average ($\bar{Y}$); this is the "explained" variation in Y_t. The denominator is the sum of squares of the deviations of the actual values of Y_t from the sample average; this is the total variation in Y_t. For example, if $R^2 = 0.90$, then 90 percent of the variation of the sample values of Y are accounted for or "explained" by the regression equation.

Applying this to an analytical situation, assume there is a positive correlation of laboratory tests to patient days. If the regression formula is applied to the forecast model, one would need only to predict patient days as the independent variable and the dependent variable of laboratory tests would follow directly. However, a further analysis of the "goodness of fit" of the regression line to the data revealed by the R^2 of 0.6981 indicates that the fit is not as good as one would like. Generally, an R^2 greater than 0.750 is adequate for projection purposes. Therefore, the forecaster should search for additional independent variables, such as patient admissions, to better explain laboratory tests.

It is important that the forecaster search for independent variables that are reasonable in explaining a dependent variable. For example, it may be that the number of patient days is directly correlated with the number of birds migrating south for the winter. However, the relationship appears to be logically unreasonable and therefore should not be used as a factor. But patient days correlated with population trends in the hospital's service area or with the number of staff physicians is a reasonable relationship and should be further explored.

Finally, the predictive value of the regression model in forecasting statistics is directly related to the predictability of the independent variable. If the independent variable can be predicted with a high degree of accuracy, the relationship is useful in the forecast of the dependent variable.

COMMUNITY MEDICAL CENTER: FORECASTING STATISTICS

Chapter 13 provided statistical projections for Community Medical Center for 1980 through the projection of revenues from operations. The projection of 117,428 patient days was based on a consensus of the administration team of the center. During the presentation of the 1980 budget to the board of directors, one director asked for a more quantifiable approach to support statistical projections. In Chapter 2, population trends for the area were presented; these may form a basis for patient-days projections utilizing regression analysis.

With this background, the reader asks for a patient-day forecast and a laboratory inpatient-procedure forecast. The controller accumulates the data in Tables 14–1 and 14–2 on historic patient days and laboratory procedures. At this point, the reader becomes directly involved in the analysis, working closely with the controller in the development of the statistical analyses of the data. This analysis should include time-series decomposition for historic patient days and regression analysis of laboratory procedures related to the independent variable of patient days.

It is essential that the reader analyze the data input in the model used. It is possible that the data are in error or that inconsistencies exist in the quantification and counting of the data. For example, the reader should review the laboratory data presented in Table 14–2 and test for reasonableness and major shifts in the data. Particularly in the laboratory area, the data may be defective due to different weightings given the data in accordance with pathological weighting mechanisms. Thus, the reader may be able to identify possible distortions in the data for the laboratory and to identify possible causes for any discrepancies.

After performing the data analysis, the reader should compare the results with the actual projections presented for the center's 1980 budget and then list the pros and cons related to the analyses and the original forecast.

Table 14-1 Community Medical Center: Historic Monthly Patient Days

Month	1977	1978	1979
January	9322	9079	10028
February	8820	8421	9627
March	9958	9034	10356
April	9527	8488	9529
May	9421	8476	9602
June	8596	9025	9747
July	9064	9546	9097
August	9254	9533	9738
September	9194	9567	9286
October	9294	9495	9740
November	8624	9316	9016
December	7467	8800	8337
Total	108541	108780	114103

Table 14-2 Community Medical Center: Historic Monthly Laboratory Procedures

Month	1977	1978	1979
January	31154	43396	53037
February	27298	40356	49055
March	35181	45332	54155
April	36507	44310	47086
May	35066	43184	49794
June	35298	46543	49759
July	46106	52349	48313
August	39621	51178	53092
September	35053	49776	49305
October	40625	46117	48310
November	35540	35658	45335
December	35607	46701	38697
Total	433056	544900	585938

Chapter 15

Cost Analysis and Rate Setting

INTRODUCTION

The forecasting of activity statistics forms the basis for the forecasting of revenues and expenses. Expenses may be forecasted in a variety of ways, including the subjective analysis of planned costs by administration and/or departmental managers, industrial engineering studies of fixed and variable costs on a detailed basis, and the use of statistical techniques such as regression analysis in the identification of fixed and variable costs on a historical experience basis. The first section of this chapter identifies cost classifications and examines the forecasting of fixed and variable costs utilizing regression analysis of historic costs.

The analysis of direct departmental costs and the identification of overhead items on a departmental basis are both important in the establishment of rates in the planning process. As we have seen, one cost allocation method is the single cost step-down utilized in the Medicare cost report. A modification of the Medicare approach is direct allocation to ancillary and patient care areas without allocation to other overhead areas. Other methods are the use of simultaneous equations, and the allocation of overhead, not as a single cost step-down, but as a double allocation of overhead areas to all areas serviced. A final cost allocation method involves the concept that planning and cost analysis should be based on weighted units of activity such as levels of patient activity. Each of these methods is discussed and illustrated in the concluding section on cost forecasting.

The concept that each department or operating area should maintain a positive cash flow after inclusion of all financial components, plus a factor for a positive rate of return, forms the basis for an expanded break-even-point analysis, which involves previous analyses of cost. Our discussion of this method utilizes cash flow analysis and discounted cash flow theories in the development of a rate setting strategy to formalize the operational aspects of the institution.

Hospital administrators should recognize that operational diversity and the vast array of services make it difficult to develop a purely flexible budget. Staffing patterns must be developed that provide for the most stable staffing to avoid layoffs in critical staffing areas, such as nursing personnel who are not easily hired in most areas of the country. Minimum levels of staffing are required to provide the best possible patient care without regard to short-term fluctuations in activity. A flexible budget is useful in the analysis of actual-versus-budget activity and constitutes a significant tool for the planning process.

COST BEHAVIOR

Cost behavior can be classified under two main headings—fixed costs and variable costs. Fixed costs can be defined as those costs that do not vary in the short term and whose volume extends over a "normal" range of activity. Short term means that all costs can be considered variable over a long enough time frame. A "normal" range of activity means that costs exhibit extreme fluctuations as activity approaches zero and as it approaches capacity. Examples of fixed costs are depreciation and interest. Variable costs can be defined as those costs that vary directly with changes in activity. Examples are film costs, which vary with the number of x-ray procedures. Costs can have both fixed and variable components. Such costs are defined as semivariable. An example is electricity or gas, which have varying rates as units of use increase. Figure 15–1 illustrates the various types of cost behavior.

ANALYZING COST

Due to the great diversity in services provided in a health care institution and the vast amount of time involved in an item-by-item cost analysis, we must seek simplifying assumptions and procedures. If we make a simplifying assumption that ignores semivariable costs, we can compare the data from (a) and (b) in Figure 15–1 to historical costs with the effects of price level changes removed to estimate the fixed and variable components of departmental costs, as shown in Figure 15–2.

Figure 15–1 Graphic Representation of Cost Behaviors

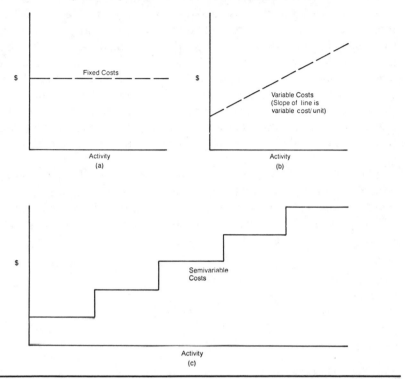

Figure 15–2 Fixed and Variable Components of Departmental Costs

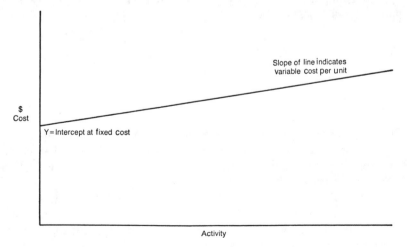

There are several methods that may be used in estimating the cost components. The easiest, but least accurate and informative, is the high-low method, based on the theory that costs will vary linearly with activity over the time horizon being considered. With this method, we can find the highest activity with its related cost and the lowest activity with its related cost. If our assumptions are correct, the incremental cost will be the variable cost associated with the increased activity. By dividing the incremental cost by the increase in activity, we determine the variable cost per unit. By multiplying the variable cost per unit and either the high or low activity and subtracting this variable component from the corresponding total cost, we find the fixed cost.

A more detailed analysis of cost behavior can be made by simply charting costs and revenues on a scattergram. By visually placing a line to "fit" the points, we can determine visually the fixed and variable components of cost. The slope of the line can be determined by examining two points on the line where the coordinates of the points are (Activity,^{1} Cost^1) and (Activity,^{2} Cost^2). The slope can be defined as:

$$\frac{(\text{Cost}^2 - \text{Cost}^1)}{(\text{Activity}^2 - \text{Activity}^1)}$$

This number is the variable cost per unit of activity. By extending the line to the Y-axis (vertical axis) where activity is zero, we find the fixed cost.

A similar but more exact way to analyze costs is the least-square-fit method by which we define a line $Y = A + B x$ where A = fixed cost, B = variable cost per unit, x = activity, and Y = cost. Thus:

$$B = \frac{n \Sigma (XY) - (\Sigma X)(\Sigma Y)}{n \Sigma X^2 - (\Sigma X)^2} \; ; A = \frac{\Sigma Y - B \Sigma X}{n}$$

The above procedures for determining fixed and variable components of total cost are valid if one assumes a consistent price level. That is, valid comparisons between activity and costs are not possible if the cost data include varying price levels.

Given current pressures to contain cost, to "market" services, and to maintain financial viability, the health care professional must know as much as possible about the costs of operation. This knowledge can then be easily translated into planning and control functions and rate setting.

To determine the required constant price level, a series of prime indexes may be used to inflate historic costs to price levels for future periods. The general format for price level computations in the inflation process is:

$$\text{Actual cost}_n \times \frac{\text{Index for future period}}{\text{Index for year n}}$$

From this, one may inflate historic data to future years' price levels and then proceed with the analysis for the computation of fixed and variable costs.

As an example of the computations involved in the above discussion, assume the data in Table 15–1 are available for the radiology department of Community Medical Center. If we apply the inflation index procedures previously described, the cost for 1973 at 53,799 procedures in 1980 dollars is:

$$\$491,526 \times \frac{174}{100} = \$855,255$$

By applying the same procedures to the other years, we have the procedures and costs in Table 15–2, stated in terms of the 1980 price level.

The next step is to project the fixed and variable components of cost through linear regression analysis, with procedures as the independent variable and cost as the dependent variable. The results of this process (outlined in detail in the previous chapter) are an equation indicating total cost for 1980 = $12,175 (procedures) + $199,576. Therefore, the total cost in 1980 based on 93,170 is $12,175 (93,170) + $199,576 = $1,333,921.

Table 15–1 Community Medical Center: Historic Costs and Indexes

Year	Procedures	Direct Cost	Index
1973	53,799	$ 491,526	100
1974	55,022	512,373	103
1975	61,872	572,101	105
1976	65,297	611,503	108
1977	73,911	694,871	112
1978	76,728	831,307	120
1979	85,694	1,090,700	157
1980	93,170		174

Table 15-2 Community Medical Center: Procedures and Adjusted Costs

Year	Procedures	Adjusted Costs
1973	53,799	$ 855,255
1974	55,022	865,562
1975	61,872	948,053
1976	65,297	985,199
1977	73,911	1,079,532
1978	76,728	1,205,395
1979	85,694	1,208,801
1980	93,170	

The inflation indexes may be derived by a detailed analysis of cost on a per-procedure basis for each department, or the published cost increase index for the medical sector by the U.S. Bureau of Labor Statistics may serve as a general measure that is useful for at least a gross analysis.

It may be argued that inflation-adjusted revenue is a better independent variable than procedures, since the more intuitively complex the procedure, the higher the per-procedure charge. For example, the charge for a CAT scan is higher than the charge for a chest x-ray. The analyst should use trial and error in determining the best set of statistics to use in the analysis.

COST ALLOCATION PROCEDURES

The objective of cost allocation is the distribution of overhead costs to the revenue-producing areas to serve as a basis for rate setting and determining the relationship of full cost to the revenues generated. There are several alternatives to the use of full cost in the analysis of cash flows as a single step-down allocation process, utilizing the readily available Medicare cost report. These include allocation of overhead only to the revenue areas with no allocation to the other general service areas, allocation of overhead to all service and revenue centers on a double allocation basis, and allocations based on the solution of a series of simultaneous equations. To illustrate these methods, the following examples will also show the single cost step-down method for comparative purposes.

In the first procedure, the allocation of overhead is made only to the revenue producing centers. The benefits of this procedure relate to the ease of computation and the fact that overhead is indeed allocated to the revenue-producing departments. A major criticism of this approach is that, in fact, service areas provide services to other service departments and the full utilization of all service areas by various revenue areas varies over the range of revenue areas.

To avoid this criticism, the single cost step-down procedure may be utilized. This procedure allocates overhead to other service areas before allocation is made to the revenue areas. However, the allocation process is based on the assumption that costs do not apply to overhead areas that are allocated first. For example, employee health and welfare may be allocated before housekeeping services. However, employee health and welfare does use housekeeping, and the allocation to employee health and welfare would not be made with the single cost step-down method.

To answer the above criticism, the double cost step-down procedure may be utilized. With this procedure, costs are allocated initially to the areas applicable before and after the cost to be allocated. Thus, in the previous example, employee health and welfare would be allocated on the first iteration to housekeeping but not on the second iteration. Therefore, this procedure only partially answers the criticism of the single step-down method.

Using a third method, the simultaneous equations model, there is full allocation to all areas of the step-down, thus providing the most accurate analysis of costs. However, this procedure can be performed only on a limited number of cost centers by manual calculation. It requires the assistance of a computer to deal with the multitude of costs and centers operating in a hospital.

RATE SETTING

Each health care institution must have a target rate of return that provides for future expansion and replacement of assets, adequate working capital, and a return to share holders. Consistently, government regulations ranging from Medicare and Medicaid to cost containment to prospective reimbursement have sought to erode capital generation for future programs. It can be easily demonstrated that operations at a break-even point will force closings and bankruptcy within the industry, leaving a large segment of the general public without adequate and critical services.

As noted earlier, the costs of functional areas include direct and indirect costs, with fixed and variable components of each type. Indirect costs generally are fixed in nature, with depreciation, administrative services, and financing expenses making up the bulk. Charting these costs by functional area, we can derive a graphic presentation of total costs, as in Figure 15–3.

Figure 15-3 Costs by Functional Area

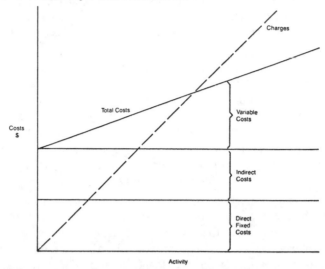

By identifying a rate of return by function, we can add this to our chart to arrive at a total requirement: total cost + return = total requirement. Charges per unit can now be set where charge (units) = variable costs + indirect costs + fixed costs, or (charge − variable costs) (units) = indirect + fixed costs. As can be seen, we can alter charges depending on variances in any one of these components. Figure 15-3 provides a graphic indication of the break-even point.

With these tools, one can plan and evaluate existing services and can justify charges based on utilization and cost behavior. Prospective reimbursement, rate review, and planning requirements can now be analyzed on a basis that eliminates the need for guesswork and subjective evaluation.

Cost benefit or present value analysis can be extended to existing and future services. By identifying the costs of services offered and the anticipated revenues from these services as they presently exist, we have the basic requirements for analyzing the effectiveness of these services. This is done through a determination of the internal rate of return of these services by finding that discount rate that will discount the future cash flows from operations back to the present time so that the present value equals capital investments as they presently exist. By adding the capital requirements for future years into these calculations, one can identify asset generations required to meet future operating needs and can identify those services that are not meeting the required rate of return.

To quantify the graphic representation of the break-even point, the following analysis is made on a simplified cash flow model: cash flow = gross revenue − direct expense − cash indirect expense − cost reimbursement percentage (gross revenue − direct expense − cash indirect expense − depreciation) − bad debt percentage (gross revenue). If we substitute into the above equation the current formula of direct cost = fixed + variable cost = fixed cost + variable cost/procedure (procedures) and then simplify, we derive the following set of equations:

If: Gross revenue = Charge/procedure × procedures,
then: Cash flow = Charge/procedure × Procedures (1 − Cost reimbursement % − bad debt %) − Fixed cost (1 − Cost reimbursement %) − Variable cost/Procedure × Procedures (1 − Cost reimbursement %) + Cost reimbursement % × Depreciation − Cash indirect expenses (1 − Cost reimbursement %).

The required cash flow is dependent on a variety of factors. Inflation expected in the future, anticipated capital requirements for the area, and a required profit margin are all related to the required cash flows from a particular area. The required cash flow should be the result of a decision made at the highest possible level of the institution, based on policies on return and practices that are appropriate to the hospital's external environment.

To illustrate, assume that the radiology department of Community Medical Center has the following additional information available for 1980:

- Depreciation: $200,000.

- Future cash-flow equipment requirements per year: $200,000/year stated in current dollars.

- Original cash investment: $1,000,000.

- Required rate of return: 7 percent.

- Required cash flow relative to initial investment: $1,000,000 (1/.07) = $70,000 (reference discount factor for infinite life = 1/required rate).

Thus, the required annual cash flow equals $200,000 + $70,000. Assume also that cost reimbursement is 52 percent and bad debt is 4 percent. If cash indirect expenses equal a net $450,000 after allocation of nonoperating revenue, we have the following computation:

$270,000 − Charge/Procedure × 93,170(1 − 52% − 4%) − $199,576 (1 − 52%) − $12.175(93,170) (1 − 52%) + 52%($200,000) − $450,000(1 − 52%).

Solving this equation, we determine that the necessary charge per procedure is equal to $24.25.

The advantages of the above analysis relate to the cost base of the charge per procedure. If a cost base has not been utilized before, the hospital should evaluate all areas of the institution and establish rates on a reasonable basis. The reason for doing this is that hospitals have historically relied on some areas of the institution to "carry" other areas of operation. In switching quickly to a cost base without a sound and systematic long-range schedule, the hospital may have difficulty justifying the dramatic increases to their service area.

COMMUNITY MEDICAL CENTER: LABORATORY COST ANALYSIS

The 1980 budget of Community Medical Center has previously been projected on a fixed basis and on an informal rate setting basis. The task for the reader at this point is to evaluate the costs of the center's laboratory as presented in Table 15-3, given the analytical methods described in the present chapter. The reader should list the pros and cons of each approach and make a critical comparison of the two proposed budgets.

Table 15-3 Community Medical Center: Laboratory Cost Analysis

Year	Procedures	Cost	Index
1971	246,012	$263,207	100
1972	271,698	291,303	104
1973	291,699	314,044	108
1974	286,538	325,646	113
1975	322,703	371,059	120
1976	349,796	411,880	126
1977	479,516	536,423	132
1978	602,230	684,890	143
1979	701,691	887,339	164
1980	718,472	X	202

Assuming the following additional information, the reader should determine the laboratory's fixed and variable costs and the appropriate charge per procedure in 1980:

- Cost reimbursement percentage: 52 percent.
- Bad debts: 4 percent.
- Depreciation: $100,000.
- Original equipment cost: $500,000.
- Required rate of return: 7 percent.
- Net cash overhead: $160,000.

Chapter 16

Financial Modeling

INTRODUCTION

A financial model is merely a quantitative description of the interrelationships of financial data, based on a system of postulates, data, and inferences presented as a mathematical description of an entity or state of affairs. In its broadest sense, a model is the presentation of abstract ideas in an observable and communicable form. Financial planning models portray financial results based on certain indicators of projected activity. Models may be certainty (definitional) or probabilistic; they may also be classified as normative or descriptive.

In this chapter, we shall be concerned with the identifying characteristics of sound financial models. In previous chapters, we examined the short-term financial plan or budget, which, in itself, is a financial planning model. Here, we will concentrate on the development of longer-range financial models through the development of pro forma financial statements similar to those presented previously.

CLASSIFICATION OF MODELS

Financial models may be certainty (descriptive) or probabilistic. A certainty model is exemplified by the accounting equation of assets = liabilities + fund balance. This accounting equation is definitional in that the equation applies regardless of the specific data elements inputted into the model. A probabilistic model is based on uncertainty, with the output of the model in the form of a probability distribution. For example, assume a distribution of input data into the model as shown in Table 16–1.These input data may be viewed in the following format of model relationships.

Table 16-1 Distribution of Input Data in a Financial Model

Market Size	Probability	% of Market	Probability	% of Sales: Material	Probability	% of Sales: Labor	Probability
100,000	.10	10	.30	40	.05	5	.05
90,000	.70	20	.30	38	.20	45	.20
80,000	.15	30	.20	35	.50	40	.20
60,000	.05	40	.10	32	.20	35	.50
		50	.10	30	.05	30	.05

Administrative Expense	Probability	Interest Rate	Probability
$5 million	.80	.080	.10
$6 million	.10	.085	.15
$4.5 million	.10	.090	.20
		.095	.30
		.100	.25

- Total assets = $20,000,000 + .10 (amount by which sales exceed $30,000,000).

- Beginning net worth = $8,000,000.

- Accounts payable = 0.5 (total assets − $16,000,000).

- Interest expense = interest rate (total assets − net worth − accounts payable).

- Earnings before deductions = (sales) − 0.48 (earnings before deductions).

- Net income = earnings before deductions − revenue deductions.

The output of this model will be a series of 7,500 elements in a probability distribution, based on the input of the series of probability distributions indicated in Table 16-1. In light of these results, it is the task of the administration to identify the most probable outcomes and the key elements that may be controlled administratively.

As noted, models may be normative or descriptive. A normative model addresses the way things should be, while a descriptive model is based on the way things are without regard to the way they should be. In health care delivery systems, it is impossible at this point to develop a normative model because of the impossibility of defining objectively good health or the services and expenditures that should be offered.

A financial model is a simplified representation of reality just as financial statements are models of the financial operations of an institution. Planning models are somewhat more difficult to evaluate than financial statements. One must have some basic criteria for evaluating planning models. Five such criteria follow.

1. The results of a good planning model must be accurate. In this regard, historical results may be compared with the model's output to verify the model's accuracy.
2. The assumptions and relationships used in the model must be reasonable. The integrity of the model must be evaluated. It is inappropriate to use nonsense relationships in the model even if the results of the past are accurate, e.g., forecasting admissions based on the number of red cars in the service area.
3. The benefits of the model must be greater than the costs of the system and the data necessary to prepare the forecast. This particularly applies to extensive models, for which the incremental cost/benefits of the system may be evaluated.
4. The model must provide useful results. The output of the model must provide information that is useful to the user and provides data that assists in the management of the institution.
5. A good model describes relationships and logical flows as a means of enhancing the decision-making process of management. Though the final results may be useful, the model's output may be based on assumptions and relationships that are known only to the administration and could be mistaken and detrimental to future operations of the organization. A model is best used when it describes to the administration the complex interrelationships that can affect the implementation and results of various decisions.

Generally, the most useful models are relatively simple and easily understandable by the user. The model should be subjected to a cost benefit analysis in that the cost of the model's operation should not exceed the resulting incremental benefits of improved managerial decision making.

For the development of a simple planning model, assume the following:

- Sales = S, which may be inputted from outside the model.
- Expense = .8(S).
- Depreciation = .10 (fixed assets$_{t-1}$).
- Net operating income (NOI) = S − expenses − depreciation.

- Interest = long term debt (LTD) × interest rate.
- Earnings before deductions (EBD) = NOI − interest.
- Deductions (D) = EBD × .48.
- Current assets (CA) = .50(S).
- Fixed assets (FA) = .60(S).
- Total assets (TA) = CA + FA
- Current liabilities (CL) = .25(S).
- Net worth (NW) = NW_{t-1} + NOI
- Long-term debt (LTD) = TA − CL − NW
- Total liabilities + NW = CL + LTD + NW

Substituting into the equation for LTD, we have the following:

$$LTD = \frac{TA - CL - NW_{t-1} \times .52(NOI)}{1 - .52i}$$

The above analysis represents a financial model based on the identification of relatively few inputs: sales, net worth$_{t-1}$, and the interest rate. The relationships developed in the model are based on the historic relationships of financial data from financial statements in previous periods. The use of simultaneous equations by substitution simplifies the model and the number of input elements.

PRO FORMA ANALYSIS

The above financial model provides the basic elements of a financial statement series of reports. By placing the data elements into the form of a set of financial statements, a series of pro forma financial statements is developed. The uses of pro forma financial statements include the following:

- identification of needed funds, based on the model's assumptions
- planning for the use of funds or income
- evaluation of the sources of funds
- evaluation of alternative decision choices
- identification of the impact of things that the institution cannot control

Pro forma financial statements can also identify the effects of a change in variables, such as the effect of sales on expenses, asset needs, and the sources of funds. The structural forecast of financial statement elements is most difficult and should therefore be subject to review by the administration for reasonableness. The benefit of pro forma analysis lies in the ability to identify the effects of uncontrollable variables, such as inflation, on the results of financial operations and on the financial position of the institution at the end of the forecasted operational period.

COMMUNITY MEDICAL CENTER: PRO FORMA FINANCIAL STATEMENTS

The pro forma financial statements for Community Medical Center presented in Chapter 11 were developed from the historic financial statements of the center. At that point, the assumptions and key indicators related to the development of the pro forma financials were summarized.

It is now the responsibility of the center's administration to evaluate the basic assumptions used in the development of the statements and to determine the key relationships of their significant areas. In the analysis of the data, the reader should address the following areas and issues:

- Are the basic utilization data valid and based on reasonable analyses of present and future circumstances?

- Are the relationships of the areas of the statement of revenues and expenses reasonable in the light of historic trends?

- Are the relationships used in the development of the balance sheet reasonable?

- What are the key areas that would affect the potential for achieving projected results?

- If the activity of patient days increases by 10 percent or decreases by 10 percent, what would be the approximate effects on the forecast?

- What effects would a 20-percent inflation rate have on the financial statements?

The answers to the above questions should be of significant concern to the reader as a center administrator who is contemplating a major expansion program for the center. In this connection, it may be helpful for the reader to refer to the material previously presented on ratio analysis.

Part V

Control

This final section deals with the control of financial operations of the institution. Control plays a prominent role in tying the other elements of the financial cycle together. It is not practical to plan, report, and take action if control of the institution's operations and the results of those operations is not maintained. Control involves the analysis and evaluation of operations in the light of planned activity and results. The mere comparing of columns of numbers without identifying the reasons for existing variances is inadequate. The comparison must be valid, in that controllable factors are identified and action is taken to correct inadequate results. The rationalization of poor results impedes the organization's efforts to deal with the future. Many times, harsh decisions and actions are required to bring the financial operations of the organization in line with expected results.

To control effectively, there must be clear objectives, policies, and procedures that are adequately communicated to those responsible for direct, daily operations. Adequate documentation and the reporting of results are essential in the control process.

In this section, Chapter 17 deals with the reporting data and analysis of planned-versus-actual financial results. The emphasis is on budget variance analysis within the operational framework of a flexible budget and the preparation of vertical and horizontal financial statement analyses on a "common size" format. Chapter 18 discusses managerial actions in the control process. Internal auditing functions and general management reporting are examined in the light of common operational problems that might hinder the uniform application of control procedures.

Chapter 17

Financial Control Analyses

INTRODUCTION

In previous chapters, in our analysis of the hospital's operations, we developed the basic components of a flexible budget through the identification of fixed and variable cost components. In practice, considerable effort is involved in the comparison and rationalization of budget-versus-actual data. Generalized rationales are often proposed for variances without regard to the dollars associated with the rationales.

In this context, the present chapter will deal first with the analysis of variances and the quantification of the reasons given for the variances. It will then examine the development of vertical or "common-size" financial statements that identify key trends in the operating results and position of the institution, without regard to inflation factors and increases in absolute quantities of the data under analysis.

VARIANCE ANALYSIS

Given available data on direct costs, indirect or overhead costs, and cost performance, we can now develop a mechanism for cost evaluation and rate setting. First, based on the fixed and variable components of cost, cost variances from a financial plan can be analyzed.

There are two basic variances to consider: cost and volume. Cost variances are related to the cost differences alone, without regard to volume differentials. We have indicated that total planned costs are defined as:

$$TC = VC/Unit \times Units + FC$$

where: TC = Total cost
VC = Variable cost
FC = Fixed cost

Given actual total cost and levels of activity, we can now define the cost variances as:

$$TC_A - VC_B (U_A) - FC_B = CV$$

where: TC_A = Actual total cost
VC_B = Variable cost planned
U_A = Actual activity
FC_B = Planned fixed cost
CV = Cost variance

The volume variance relates to the coverage of fixed costs by anticipated-versus-actual activity levels. Therefore, we determine planned fixed cost per planned unit and multiply this by the difference between actual activity and planned activity to yield the volume variance.

The hospital thus has a method for identifying and controlling costs of services that are planned on a flexible basis with units of service, not on a fixed "budget," which hides variances with changes in activity levels. By dividing the institution into functional areas, one can easily extrapolate these methods to new services with identifiable elements of costs, such as staffing, as fixed and variable units, thus eliminating the need for a high level of fixed costs that may or may not vary logically with unit changes in activity.

In the radiology area of Community Medical Center, we saw in Chapter 15 that the direct fixed budgeted cost was $199,576 and the budgeted variable cost per unit was $12,175. The budgeted number of procedures was 93,170. Assume that the actual total expense was $1,500,000, with a volume of 95,000 procedures. Using simple nonstandard variance analysis, the reader should now be able to compute the controllable and volume variances for the radiology area.

VERTICAL AND HORIZONTAL ANALYSIS

It is difficult to identify internal relationships by utilizing the absolute numbers that make up the financial statements. To identify these relationships more clearly, it is possible to perform vertical or common-size analysis on the data elements in the financial statements. The procedures are relatively simple, in that a base number is chosen and the rest of the elements in the statement are shown as a percentage of the base number.

The advantages of common-size analysis is in the capability to identify internal relationship trends in the financial statements. Note that in the composition of the assets section of the balance sheet of Community Medical Center, trends between two years indicated the financing of significant capital acquisition from internally generated funds. This was evidenced by a shift of board-designated funds from 9.44 percent of total assets in 1978 to 5.99 percent in 1979.

In this analysis, there is no evidence of major shifts in the liabilities of the institution that might offset the financial requirements placed on the investments of the institution. The positive aspects of the analysis stem from the elimination of absolute numbers, which managerially are not easily compared.

In the statement of revenues and expenses, there is a shift toward increased revenue deductions and increased salaries relative to other areas of the expense category. Again it is difficult to judge the positive and/or negative aspects of such shifts without knowledge of the administration's plans for the composition movement. Based on common-size analysis, however, it is easy for the administration to deal with the establishment of required trends and shifts in the composition of the components of the financial statements, if only on an intuitive level.

Horizontal analysis, which will not be examined in detail here, is merely the computation of the percentages of change between time periods for various components of the financial statements.

At this point, the reader should perform the vertical-analysis computations for the financials presented in Chapter 2 for the Community Medical Center. The same basic analysis can be made utilizing horizontal-analysis procedures. In this case, significant shifts in the components of the financial statements may be identified by the percentage of change computed for the components. The disadvantage of this approach, it should be noted, is that the size of the components being compared does have direct effect on the size of the variation. An increase of one dollar on a two-dollar item yields a 50 percent increase, which has little relevance considering the absolute size of the amounts being compared.

COMMUNITY MEDICAL CENTER: VERTICAL ANALYSIS

As a final exercise, the reader should analyze the pro forma financial statements presented for Community Medical Center in Chapter 16, utilizing the vertical or common-size analytical technique. In this analysis, the reader should develop key indicators of the trends in the financial statements and develop at least subjective requirements for the future in areas such as liquidity, salaries, and so on.

Chapter 18

Managerial Aspects of Financial Control

INTRODUCTION

In this final chapter, the material presented in previous chapters is placed in proper perspective within the management area of the hospital. The various phases of the financial cycle previously examined are relatively meaningless unless they are guided by the managerial philosophy of the organization. The hospital administration must be in constant touch with the financial operations of the organization and should take direct responsibility for the overall direction of its fiscal affairs.

Our purpose at this point is to identify the key managerial elements in the control of financial operations. Our starting point is an examination of internal auditing, not only from a financial standpoint but also from the standpoint of an operational audit function within the organization. This function deals with the extent of overall adherence to the policies and procedures established by the administration and with the hospital's dedication to the improvement of overall organizational productivity and patient care.

Based on this examination, the key elements necessary to the development of sound policies and procedures in the fiscal operation of the organization can be identified. Only by establishing both the plans and the processes by which the plans will be achieved will the administration of the hospital have a guide in the control of activities conducted by diverse individuals in the organization. The logical follow-up to this analysis is an examination of the concept of management by objectives (MBO). Key elements of an MBO system are explored, and the relationship of MBO to financial control is discussed. Finally, the testing and specific applications of the concepts and methods developed throughout the previous discussions will be summarized.

INTERNAL AUDITING

The internal audit function is illustrated by the actions of an accountant who reconciles bank statements, counts cash, and verifies account balances with an eye toward the identification of fraud or theft. As a general proposition, it may be said that the internal audit, though initially concerned with adherence to the financial control objectives established by the organization, is a useful function for the control of all policies and operations of the institution in line with policy guidelines established by the hospital administration.

Internal auditing is in the domain of operational auditing, by which a review is made of all existing policies and procedures and of actual operations in effect to ensure that they are in accordance with the wishes of the governing body of the institution. For example, if the internal auditor wants to verify the distribution of payroll checks, the primary goal of the verification is to ensure that only authorized personnel are receiving paychecks. However, the real benefit of such an examination derives from the auditor's ability to investigate as well other areas of personnel administration, such as position control, the scheduling of personnel, and the use of overtime rather than the adjusting of schedules. In this context, the auditor is no longer concerned primarily with the distribution of paychecks but with the overall management of positions and the effective, productive utilization of personnel.

It is essential that the hospital's administration fully endorse this concept and communicate it to all managers in the organization. The potential benefits of the operational audit are limited when the manager in the area under audit feels threatened by the process. Thus, all audit procedures and guidelines should be approved by the hospital administration and also by the department head being audited. Also, of course, the operational auditor must be qualified, knowledgeable of the organization, and aware that the auditing job is to assist rather than condemn.

DEVELOPMENT OF POLICIES AND PROCEDURES

The basis for control is the development and communication of policies and procedures in conjunction with the administration of the institution. It is impossible to manage effectively if the goals and expectations of management are not known by those responsible for direct action. Thus, policies and procedures must be developed to include at least the following elements:

- All policies and procedures should be clear, concise, and easily understood by those responsible for their administration.

- Important policies should be communicated in writing and acknowledged by the appropriate persons in the organization.

- Attainable and measurable guidelines must be associated with the policies. For example, an instruction that receivables should be reduced is not enough. The instruction should require that the days in receivables are to be reduced by two days by the end of the year; this is more specific, and the attainment of the goal is measurable.

- Goals, policies, and procedures should be jointly developed by those responsible for their administration. In this way, the goals, policies, and procedures are not dictated but are rather the result of communication between levels of management.

- The administration should review adherence to policies and procedures on a timely basis, maintaining continuous communication with managers responsible for their implementation.

- The administrator should remember that, even in an area as abstract as finance, the hospital administration is responsible for overall direction of the area's operation.

All of the above are incorporated in a management process known as management by objectives (MBO). This process requires the establishment of specific and measurable goals jointly between upper and lower levels of management. The manager is responsible for progress within a set time frame and is required to maintain communication with higher management regarding progress and the general state of affairs in the area under scrutiny. It is essential that the MBO process include financial goals and require the establishment of a plan and the evaluation of actual performance against the plan. Such direct involvement identifies areas that require administrative action and in which there may be errors in the assumptions of the plan. This ties in closely with the requirements of financial planning and the analysis of variances.

SUMMARY

In implementing the methods and concepts presented in the previous chapters, it should be remembered that there are no fixed formulas for the effective management of fiscal operations in a health care institution. There are only general guidelines and management theory to determine the elements in the financial cycle of reporting, planning, action, and control.

The general format of the basic set of financials, together with the key elements of their development, should in practice be adjusted and questioned, keeping in mind the goal of improved management reporting. Conceivably, a circumstance could arise where the daily cash flow is managerially more important than the daily statements of revenue and expense. The administrator is the one who must direct the development of managerially useful report information. Without the administrator's involvement, the financial manager will not be able to provide information that is useful to overall management.

In monitoring current issues in the health care environment and identifying the key elements in the internal management of the financial organization, it is essential to have an organizational structure that is flexible enough to be reactive, with administrators who are aware of the hospital's environmental conditions and who can address issues on an offensive rather than defensive basis.

The financial management of the health care organization must be based on a plan that addresses future issues in the institution and its dealings with the external environment. The financial planning section of the cycle addresses this aspect specifically. Furthermore, the financial plan must be based on a realistic evaluation of current and projected circumstances in the organization. The plan should include participation by as many segments of the hospital's population as possible. In this context, the hospital must generate funds to provide for the future expansion of services and the provision of constantly improved patient care. Thus, the financial plan must incorporate an adequate rate of return in the light of cost and inflation aspects of the environment and the overall plans of the institution.

Control, the final element of the financial cycle, begins with a commitment by the administration of the hospital to evaluate its position on an ongoing and realistic basis. Continuous evaluation of and adherence to established policies and procedures are essential to ensure improved productivity in line with the organization's goals and objectives. In short, the hospital's primary goal must be always to provide the best possible care to its patients within the constraints of available funds. Those constraints can be dealt with effectively as long as the controls of the hospital's financial operations remain the primary concern of the administration.

Index

Note: Italicized page numbers indicate tables.

About the Author

JERRY L. BOLANDIS, M.B.A., C.P.A., has been associated with St. Elizabeth Medical Center, Granite City, Illinois, since January, 1973 and is presently Controller of that 400-bed facility. He has a B.A. in mathematics and an M.B.A. from Southern Illinois University in Edwardsville. He is presently working toward a Ph.D. in finance at St. Louis University. Since 1977, he has been an instructor of finance in the Department of Hospital and Health Care Administration at St. Louis University.

Mr. Bolandis has published articles in *Hospital Financial Management* and has given presentations on financial management to members of the Hospital Financial Management Association (HFMA) and to the American College of Nursing Home Administrators. He is a senior member of the HFMA. He is also vice-president and treasurer of Providence Management and Marketing Services, a consulting firm.

Mr. Bolandis resides with his wife Janet and three children, Beth, Matthew, and Brooke, in Granite City, Illinois.